PRAISE FOR

The Low-Fat Lifestyle

If you are looking for a new tool to help you live life to the fullest, look
no further. Amy Nappa has provided a practical resource for all of us who
want to maximize our physical, emotional, and spiritual well-being. *The
Low-Fat Lifestyle* is sensible, realistic, and thoroughly biblical. Read this
book and rejuvenate your life!

> —DRS. LES AND LESLIE PARROTT, authors of *Becoming
> Soul Mates*

The Low-Fat Lifestyle is an inspirational guide for those striving to make
healthier choices in their daily lives. Amy Nappa teaches us how to nurture our bodies—and souls—with low-fat foods. The recipes are particularly helpful!

> —CATHERINE M. SURIANO, M.D.

As the wife of a husband with a genetic predisposition to heart disease, I
applaud Amy Nappa's practical and personable approach to implementing sensible low-fat meal planning. But as a woman whose home is
weighed down by an overload of stuff and whose schedule is often bloated
with overcommitments, I really *need* Amy's gentle reminder that "low-fat"
applies to other areas of life as well: my time, my money, my home, my
relationship with God. Amy's wholistic approach in *The Low-Fat Lifestyle*
is refreshing and wonderful!

> —JANE JOHNSON STRUCK, editor, *Today's Christian Woman*

Amy Nappa offers us a fine prescription for "temple tending." *The Low-Fat Lifestyle* is rich in practical detail that will sustain us for a lifetime.

—DIANE M. KOMP, M.D., author of *Breakfast for the Heart*

Amy Nappa's book is a practical guide to reducing the fat in your life—body, soul, and spirit. Insightful and well researched, this is information I can highly recommend to my patients! Anyone interested in trimming all types of "fat" from life would certainly benefit from reading *The Low-Fat Lifestyle*.

—EDWIN RISENHOOVER, M.D.

A no-fad, common-sense approach to living a healthy lifestyle that is do-able without a lot of hassle and expense. Kudos to Amy Nappa for offering a simple, practical approach to eating well, feeling good, and keeping spiritually, financially, and emotionally fit.

—CINDY CROSBY, author of *Waiting for Morning*, and free-lance editor for *Publishers Weekly, Christian Retailing,* and *Today's Christian Woman*

This book is about "more," not "less"! Amy Nappa not only inspires but equips the reader to embrace a life that is rich and full in every way. Don't miss learning how to sort the "stones and rice" in your life!

—SANDY LYNAM CLOUGH, author of *When You Don't Know What to Say*

the Low-Fat Lifestyle

the Low-Fat Lifestyle

AMY NAPPA

Optimum Health

for Body, Soul,

and Spirit

WATERBROOK
PRESS

THE LOW-FAT LIFESTYLE
PUBLISHED BY WATERBROOK PRESS
2375 Telstar Drive, Suite 160
Colorado Springs, Colorado 80920
A division of Random House, Inc.

This book is not intended replace the medical advice of a trained medical professional. Readers are advised to consult a physician or other qualified health-care professional regarding treatment of their medical problems. The author and publisher specifically disclaim liability, loss, or risk, personal or otherwise, which is incurred as a consequence, directly or indirectly, of the use or application of any of the contents of this book.

All Scripture quotations, unless otherwise indicated, are taken from the *Holy Bible, New International Version®*. NIV®. Copyright © 1973, 1978, 1984 by International Bible Society. Used by permission of Zondervan Publishing House. All rights reserved. Scripture quotations marked (NCV) are taken from *The Holy Bible, New Century Version*, copyright © 1987, 1988, 1991 by Word Publishing, Nashville, TN 37214. Used by permission. Scripture quotations marked (NKJV) are taken from the *New King James Version*. Copyright © 1982 by Thomas Nelson, Inc. Used by permission. All rights reserved. Scripture quotations marked (NASB) are taken from the *New American Standard Bible®* (NASB). © Copyright The Lockman Foundation 1960, 1962, 1963, 1968, 1971, 1972, 1973, 1975, 1977, 1995. Used by permission. (www.Lockman.org). Scripture quotations marked (KJV) are taken from the *King James Version*.

Names in some anecdotes and stories have been changed to protect the identities of the persons involved.

ISBN 1-57856-631-2

Library of Congress Cataloging-in-Publication Data
Nappa, Amy, 1963–
  The low-fat lifestyle : optimum health for body, soul, and spirit / Amy Nappa.—1st ed.
    p. cm.
  Includes bibliographical references and index.
  ISBN 1-57856-631-2
  1. Christian life. 2. Low-fat diet. I. Title.
BV4596.D53 N37 2002
613.2'84—dc21

                                                            2002013188

Printed in the United States of America
2002—First Edition

10 9 8 7 6 5 4 3 2 1

For Mike,
who fills my life
with the low-fat delights of
love and laughter

Contents

Part One: The Low-Fat Body

Part Two: The Low-Fat Soul

Part Three: The Low-Fat Spirit

Acknowledgments

As is always the case in a work like this, I owe a debt of gratitude to many people for their help and support during the creation of this book.

First, to my wonderful editor, Dan Benson, whose vision and determination brought this book into being. (Dan, I hope we do a dozen more books together!) And to Keith Wall and Jennifer Lonas for their excellent editorial contributions as well.

To my son, Tony, and my sister, Annette, who never blinked and never backed away from the table no matter what new recipe I tried out during family dinners.

To Tom and Jana Tyrrell and all my dear friends (this includes you, Kay!) in our church Life Group. You all prayed me through this project, and I'm forever thankful for your friendship.

Last, but certainly not least, I'm grateful to Jesus Christ, who first showed me that this life he gave is meant to be lived—and lived to the fullest!

CREED OF THE LOW-FAT LIFESTYLE

Daily I will fill my life with an abundance
of that which is healthy, so that I will
no longer need—or eventually even want—
that which is unhealthy.

Let's Make a Promise

I came to give life—life in all its fullness.

—JESUS CHRIST (JOHN 10:10, NCV)

In the summer of 2000, I was enjoying a week of sun, surf, and sand on Catalina Island with my son and parents when I got the call. It was my husband, Mike, and he had news I'd never expected to hear.

"My body isn't processing fat properly," he told me. "I have fatty deposits on my liver, and that's a dangerous thing. I have to change the way I eat. Today. Forever. Otherwise the doctor predicts I'll have heart disease, liver disease, diabetes, or any combination of these within the next ten years."

"What?" I was shocked at this sudden news. I already knew that Mike had a chronic digestive disorder, and we'd adjusted to his regimen of medicines. I knew that a routine medical exam for an insurance policy had raised a red flag about his liver. And I knew Mike would be going to the doctor to double-check the results while I vacationed.

But I didn't know that fat was literally killing his body from the inside out. And I didn't know how much our lifestyle was about to change.

Let me make one thing clear. Mike was not overweight. Sure, at that time he could have stood to lose five or ten pounds, but apart from his chronic digestive disorder, he was in good physical shape. Based on his looks, no one would have suggested he needed to diet. Mike and I both had no reason to think we were at risk for any disease, so we ate what we liked. In fact, we ate a fairly balanced diet that included fruits, vegetables, and the other recommended food groups. What I didn't understand was how much fat we were consuming in the process. Cheese, meat, potato chips, mayonnaise, chocolate, pies—and that was just for starters!

By the time I got home from my seaside vacation, Mike had already read as much literature on low-fat eating as he could get his hands on. We went to the grocery store and began reading labels—it was an eye-opening experience. We were both surprised to learn how much fat we'd been consuming day after day, and we were ready to do something about it.

That was the beginning of the Low-Fat Lifestyle for our family.

REDUCING "FAT" IN OTHER AREAS OF LIFE

As I learned about the benefits of a diet of low-fat foods, I began to consider that the Low-Fat Lifestyle might be about far more than healthful eating. Taking fat out of my diet left more room for healthful foods. So why wouldn't the same be true in every other area of my life? If I cut the "fat" from my career, there would be more room for growth. If I cut the "fat" from my family life, there would be more time for us to enjoy each other. If I cut the "fat" from my spiritual life, I would be able to know God more fully.

I considered other aspects of life: my finances, social life, household chores, and so on. The concept of cutting out the so-called fats and filling up on goodness in all areas of life—body, soul, and spirit—made more and more sense!

I said earlier that Mike did not look physically unfit when we learned about what was happening with his body. Yet the truth was that he was hurting himself with his diet. I realized that every area of our lives needed a closer look. Things that appeared to be fine on the surface might actually be damaging. No area of life would go untouched. Health. Family. Career. Finances. Friendships. Spiritual life. All could be improved using the principles of the Low-Fat Lifestyle. I realized that when we fill our body, soul, and spirit with fat and other junk, there's little room left for anything good. Sure, we're "eating," but instead of nourishing ourselves, we end up starving ourselves. We may look healthy and feel full, but we're never nurtured, and we fail to thrive physically, mentally, or spiritually.

Jesus said, "I have come that they may have life, and have it to the full" (John 10:10). That promise is the basis for the Low-Fat Lifestyle. You see, Christ never intended to rob us of pleasure or to transform our lives into daily drudgery. Yet sometimes—too often, really—we act as if he wants to keep us from having fun.

Read Jesus' words again: "I have come that they may have life, and have it *to the full*" (emphasis added).

Do you see it? Jesus wants our lives to be *full. Full* of goodness. *Full* of love. *Full* of joy, peace, truth, strength, and more. He's not talking only about our eating. He's talking about *everything* in our lives—body, soul, and spirit. But if we're filling up our homes, our careers, our pockets, and our hearts with busyness, lies, hate, anger, indifference, and other "fatty items," we leave precious little room for Jesus to fill our lives.

That brings me to the reason for this book—and the reason (I hope) you're reading it. If you're like me, you probably feel that it's time we reclaimed our right to a full, Christ-focused life. And that's what the Low-Fat Lifestyle is all about. It's about cutting out the unhealthy fat of life and filling our lives instead with health and God's goodness. It's about living a fulfilling lifestyle that goes by the following creed:

> *Daily I will fill my life with an abundance of that which is healthy,*
> *so that I will no longer need—or eventually even want—*
> *that which is unhealthy.*

WHAT THE LOW-FAT LIFESTYLE IS NOT

Notice that our creed doesn't say, "I will deprive myself until I'm miserable" or "I will make myself suffer so that, hopefully, I'll be healthier." That's not "life to the full"!

In fact, let's clear up what the Low-Fat Lifestyle is *not*.

It's not punishment for being out of shape physically, mentally, or spiritually. Instead, it's a reward. When we don't take care of ourselves—our bodies, our daily activities, and our spiritual growth—then we're truly punishing ourselves. Let's instead reward ourselves with the goodness God has made available to us.

It's not a chore to be tolerated or endured. Taking care of ourselves in every aspect of life can be exciting and amazing. Leave behind the idea that "low-fat" means boring and tasteless. Instead, think of this change as an adventure in which you don't know what wonderful surprise will be revealed as you round each corner.

It's not a quick fix. In fact, the Low-Fat Lifestyle represents a *lifestyle* change. This isn't a fad diet or a get-your-prayers-answered-quick scheme. When you embrace this lifestyle, you embrace it from today to forever, and believe it or not, it won't be long until you won't even *want* to go back to the junk with which you used to fill your life. You'll feel too good to do that.

It's not a list of "no-no's." None of us wants to always be saying, "I can't eat that and I can't watch that and I can't listen to that and I can't go there." We want to say, "I can do it all and have it all!" With the Low-Fat Lifestyle, you'll find yourself saying yes more than ever. Yes to good nutrition. Yes to peace of mind. Yes to your family. Yes to joy. Yes to God.

TOO GOOD TO BE TRUE?

Sound too good to be true? It's not! As Christians, we have access to the best in life because we have access to Jesus Christ and the fullness of life he offers. You *can* fill your body with health. You *can* saturate your soul with joy and peace. You *can* soak your spirit with the presence of the God who loves you and gave his all for you. And you can start today.

So what do you say? Are you ready to join me in the adventure of the Low-Fat Lifestyle? Then read on and let's discover how to fill our lives with all the goodness God has in store.

PART ONE

The Low-Fat Body

The Low-Fat Lifestyle Starts Today!

But encourage each other every day while it is "today." Help each other so none of you will become hardened because sin has tricked you.

—HEBREWS 3:13 (NCV)

When we got the news that Mike had to significantly lower the amount of fat he consumed, we had to make changes immediately. There was no "grace period" for reversing the damaging effects that decades of fat consumption had wreaked on his body. We grabbed as many books and articles as we could to learn about how to fill his body with what it needed.

Interestingly enough, the more I read about the changes Mike had to make, the more I wanted to make changes in the way I was eating. I quickly learned how much fat I was dumping into my body, and I wanted to stop. But how? It's one thing to optimistically say, "I'm going to change my lifestyle." It's quite another thing to actually *do* it.

So let's begin by approaching the Low-Fat Lifestyle realistically and consider *why* we even want to change. Next we'll focus on building a healthier body by reducing the fat we consume. Then in Parts 2 and 3 we'll extend our low-fat metaphor to building a healthier soul and spirit.

THE BENEFITS OF LOW-FAT EATING

What are the benefits of low-fat eating? I'm neither a doctor nor a professional nutritionist, yet it's been easy for me to research the stacks of books, articles, and studies on the importance and benefits of low-fat eating. I won't go into all the medical data here, but if you're really interested, you can check into the resources listed in the appendix. For now, to get us moving in the right direction, let's just focus on the well-known facts.

No More "Diets"

The first benefit of this positive change is that it's *not* a diet. When we say we're "on a diet," we tend to think of our changed eating habits as temporary. We think we'll count calories or eat only certain foods until we've achieved our ideal weight, then we'll return to our old eating habits. This kind of sporadic dieting actually means we're more likely to gain weight again…and become even more discouraged than before.

So the first step to a Low-Fat Lifestyle is this: *Forget the idea of being on a diet.* Instead, determine to cheerfully say, "I'm permanently changing my eating habits." (Hey, it's not called a *lifestyle* for nothing!) No more diet means no more of the up-and-down roller coaster of losing weight only to gain it all back.

It's the old tortoise-and-hare philosophy. Instead of following diet-fad "rabbits" that take off fast only to stall before finishing last in the race, we choose the slow-and-steady tortoise approach. Day in and day out, we do the little things, making healthy choices until we don't need—or even want—unhealthy foods. Before long, like that victorious slowpoke of a turtle, we, too, will cross that finish line in first place—and be empowered by healthy habits to keep finishing first in the race of life.

Weight Loss

The second and most obvious benefit of the Low-Fat Lifestyle is weight loss. Of course, the primary goal of eating less fat is to enjoy better health, but a side benefit of filling your plate with healthy foods is that you'll start dropping unwanted pounds.

This is not to condemn or lay guilt trips on people who are overweight. Some people say, "I'm heavy, and I'm at peace with that." God does love us all, no matter how thick or thin we are. But being overweight is tough on our bodies. Carrying around extra pounds strains our muscles, bones, and organs in many ways.

When we lighten the load our bodies carry, we move toward peak physical performance, a by-product of this lifestyle change. In fact, my husband dropped more than thirty pounds during the first six months of living the Low-Fat Lifestyle. After he reached his body's ideal weight, this fat-reducing lifestyle has enabled him to keep those pounds off and maintain a consistent body weight that looks good and feels good to him.

Increased Energy

Because of his chronic health condition, Mike had been unable to volunteer or participate in many activities for several years. He simply didn't have the strength and couldn't count on his body to cooperate. But within four months of cutting his fat intake, Mike was coaching our son's basketball team. Undoubtedly, eating less fat boosted his energy level.

Of course, when you think about it, that's just common sense. The thirty pounds Mike lost is about as much as my preschool-age niece weighs, and it's no big deal for Mike to carry Brianna around on his shoulders for a short while. But if he were to carry her for an hour, he would feel tired. Imagine if Mike had to lug her around all the time—that extra thirty pounds pressing on him every time he stood up, sat down, walked around the mall, or mowed the lawn. No wonder he was tired! You and I would be too.

Now imagine the difference if, after years of carrying the weight of this little girl with him wherever he went, Mike suddenly discovered that Brianna could walk on her own. What if he set her down and let her stroll beside him instead of bearing her weight himself? He'd feel the difference right away. He'd have more energy and less pain and exhaustion. That's *exactly* how he feels. And so will you after living out the Low-Fat Lifestyle and losing unwanted pounds.

Better Health—Inside and Out

Physicians tell us that consuming less fat lowers our risk of heart disease, diabetes, and cancer. We often scowl at people who smoke or drink excessive amounts of alcohol, thinking, *She's giving herself cancer* or *He's drinking himself into the grave*. Yet how often do we make those comments while we're scarfing down a quarter-pound hamburger and fries, failing to recognize that the fat we're eating does significant damage to our own bodies? In fact, former Surgeon General Dr. David Satcher reported that three hundred thousand Americans die each year from conditions caused or worsened by being overweight.[1] These are preventable deaths!

Poor health costs us money, too. And if you're like me, you don't want to spend money on doctor's bills. One estimate shows that diseases related to poor eating habits cost Americans more than $250 billion each year in medical expenses and days missed at work.[2] Another study reports, "In 4 of the 10 leading causes of death for this country, poor diet and lack of physical activities are significant contributing factors."[3]

When it comes to our health and eating habits, we are often like the person the apostle James described in his New Testament book: "A double-minded man, unstable in all he does" (1:8). We eat a Twinkie with a diet Coke. We gorge ourselves on chicken-fried steak with onion rings, then we order low-fat frozen yogurt for dessert. It would be funny if it weren't so true.

With the Low-Fat Lifestyle we don't have to be mixed up about our health anymore. We can enjoy healthful eating and improved physical vitality as a result.

I have to tell you that when Mike first heard the news that his health was in jeopardy, he was tempted to give up, to shrug and say, "Well, if I've got ten years left, I'll just indulge myself and enjoy it." But that didn't last long, because Mike soon realized two things. First, living out even ten years in poor health just wouldn't be enjoyable. It certainly wouldn't have been the kind of abundant life Jesus promised. Mike's real choice was between living out ten years in increasingly poorer health or living out a longer lifespan in increasingly better (and more enjoyable) health. Looking at it that way, the choice was simple.

Second, Mike chose to pursue better health for the sake of our son, Tony. Mike realized that his health affects more than just himself; it has a big influence on everyone who loves him. Of course, that includes me, but when it came down to brass tacks, it was our young son who provided motivation for Mike. Having grown up without a father himself, Mike told me, "I'm going to do all I can to improve my health because Tony deserves to have a dad around as long as possible."

Your family and friends also deserve the joy of having you in their lives. By implementing a low-fat strategy, you, too, will improve your health and allow those loved ones countless more opportunities to share life with the irreplaceable you.

More Joy

If you weigh less, look better, feel better, and have more energy, you can't help but enjoy a happier, more rewarding life. You'll have more time, energy, and motivation to actively pursue and experience that "life to the fullest" our Lord has promised. (More on this later.)

These are just a few of the physical benefits of the Low-Fat Lifestyle, and you can experience them all plus a great many more that you will discover as you enjoy your healthy new habits.

HOW MUCH FAT DO YOU ACTUALLY NEED?

The next step to living a Low-Fat Lifestyle is figuring out how much fat you actually need. Not *want*, but *need*. The Low-Fat Lifestyle doesn't insist that you deprive yourself of any foods or nutrients that your body needs. Many fad diets encourage us to load up on one kind of food and exclude others. Other diet programs allow us only a certain number of calories per day. Sure, these can help us lose weight, but most often they leave us feeling hungry and deprived.

Good news! The Low-Fat Lifestyle allows plenty of food while providing the amount of fat our bodies require.

Most Americans are taking in 40 percent or more of their calories from fat.[4] Nutritionists and experts from many national organizations advise that between 20 and 30 percent of our calories should come from fat, with less than 10 percent as saturated fat. Many diet systems rely on the 30 percent figure.[5] (These diet programs also generally allow you smaller portions of the fatty foods you're already eating, which usually leaves you feeling hungry.) Recommendations aside, we truly *need* to take in only between 4 and 6 percent of our calories from fat.[6]

So how much fat should *you* consume? It's a good idea to talk to your doctor before you begin any change of diet, so you may want to start there.

For our purposes here, we want to make sure we provide the fat our bodies need, so let's agree that getting 10 percent of our calories from fat will be the ideal. To make it easy for you to figure how many fat grams you need to meet this goal, look at Charts A and B at the end of this chapter. Chart A will help you determine how much you should weigh according to your height and body frame. Insurance companies and medical groups create weight charts to give people a general idea of how much they should weigh. Such charts may vary by a few pounds depending upon who created them. They also don't take every factor into consideration, so they may be inaccurate in some cases (such as for pregnant women or for those involved in serious weightlifting). Your doctor can consider all your health and age factors and give you a more accurate weight goal, but for our purposes, Chart A will give you a general idea of how much you should weigh. For example, let's pretend we have a friend named Jennie who is 5 feet 3 inches tall and has a small frame. According to Chart A, she should weigh somewhere between 111 and 124 pounds.

Next, take your appropriate weight and find the corresponding number on Chart B. The fat grams recommended on this chart will allow for 10 percent of your calories to come from fat. This lifestyle change can meet your nutritional needs. For Jennie, 120 pounds is in the middle of her range, so she would need approximately 20 grams of fat per day to maintain good health.

I realize, however, that not everyone will be ready to make this much of a change. So here's a mathematical formula to help you figure out how many grams of fat you should have each day. Grab a calculator—it's easy!

Begin with your appropriate weight from Chart A. Take this number and multiply it by 15. This will tell you how many calories you need each day. For example, Jennie would like to weigh 120 pounds, so she would multiple this weight by 15.

$$120 \text{ x } 15 = 1,800 \text{ calories a day}$$

Next, you'll figure the percentage of fat you'll consume in grams. Multiply the calories you need by your goal percentage. Let's say Jennie has decided that reducing her fat intake to 20 percent is a more realistic goal for her than 10 percent. So she would first multiply her calorie needs by .20.

$$1800 \text{ x } .20 = 360$$

She would then divide this result by 9, since there are 9 calories in 1 gram of fat.

$$360 \div 9 = 40 \text{ grams of fat a day for Jennie}$$

This simple formula can help you set intermittent goals if you'd like to move into the Low-Fat Lifestyle more gradually. No matter what your goal, think of it as the "budget amount" you have available to spend each day. This gives you more freedom in making choices. You can choose to spend your daily fat allotment on a small amount of fatty foods, or you can spend it on an abundant amount of healthful foods. The choice is yours.

MORE GOOD NEWS

This leads us to more good news. Eating less fat actually allows you to eat more food. I know it doesn't seem to add up at first, but fat has more calories per gram than proteins and carbohydrates. I saw this principle in action recently when I was having dinner with my father. Dad is learning the Low-Fat Lifestyle, and I was helping him calculate how much fat he was eating in that meal. He was eating a soy-and-vegetable burger along with a spicy side dish of Spanish rice and black beans.

"You've got about five grams of fat there, Dad," I explained.

Since his plate was full of food, he was amazed. Then I went over to the counter and picked up two Oreo cookies.

"Two of these have seven grams of fat," I told him. "So you can eat that whole plate of food for dinner or these two cookies. Which do you want?"

It wasn't a matter of counting calories. Rather, by focusing on grams of fat and sticking to the recommended serving size, Dad could eat his fill, get plenty of the nutrients his body needed, and never feel deprived—all while losing weight.

HOW MUCH FAT ARE YOU CURRENTLY EATING?

Now that you know how much fat you need, it's time to find out how much you're currently eating. This takes a little practice and discipline, but it's not hard. It comes down to reading labels and writing down how many grams of fat you consume in a day.

By law, all prepackaged foods must include information about how much fat is in each serving. For example, a box of apple-and-cinnamon-flavored oatmeal in my cupboard tells me that one serving has 1.5 grams of fat. A serving in this case is one pouch of oatmeal. Not too tricky. A can of soup says it has 3 grams of fat per serving. In this case a serving is one cup, which means I'll need to measure out a cup of the soup instead of just digging in.

The fat content for foods that are not labeled can be found through Internet sites and books available at your local library or bookstore. I've included a few at the end of the book that I think are helpful. Chapters 3 and 4 will provide you with further information on how to read labels and what to do when you eat out. So pick up a small notepad, and each time you eat, jot down how many grams of fat you're consuming. Do this for a week, and by then you'll know where you're getting your fat.

FORMULATE A PLAN—AND RECRUIT A FRIEND

Once you see how much fat you *need* and how much you're actually taking in, you can start deciding what foods to replace in your eating plan. The first two weeks are the hardest, so ask a friend to help you stay accountable—especially during this transition time. Let's face it: Fat tastes good. In fact, not long ago Frito-Lay actually added more fat to their chips just to make them taste better![7] But when you tell people about your commitment, they'll help you stick to your plan. (And they might even join you.)

A friend whom I see often has changed her eating habits to help her lose more than one hundred pounds. I check with her regularly to see how she's doing. When I've seen doughnuts on the coffee cart, I encourage her to avoid temptation by taking the long route to the copier. I cheer her on when she skips the pork chops and eats foods that are rich in nutrients and low in fat.

It takes a couple weeks for your taste buds to adjust to less fat, but they *will* adjust, so be patient. After a few weeks of eating low-fat and no-fat foods, fatty foods will suddenly seem downright disgusting. Your body will adjust to having less fat too and won't appreciate fatty meals. For more than two years, our family has not been eating red meat, and when I recently had a fatty hamburger with a friend, I became physically sick within three hours. My body was telling me it didn't want that junk!

The action plan for you right now is to use the steps that were mentioned earlier in the chapter to determine how much fat you need. Then begin writing down how much fat you're eating.

After a week of tracking your fat intake, it'll be time to start choosing foods that will help you meet your goal. That's where the following chapters will really come in handy. But for now, tell a friend what you're doing, and let's get started on the Low-Fat Lifestyle today!

Ideal Weight by Height and Frame Size[8]

Height		Small Frame		Medium Frame		Large Frame	
Men	Women	Men	Women	Men	Women	Men	Women
5'2"	4'10"	128–134	100–110	131–141	108–120	138–150	117–131
5'3"	4'11"	130–136	101–112	133–143	110–123	140–154	119–134
5'4"	5'0"	132–138	103–115	135–145	112–126	142–156	121–137
5'5"	5'1"	134–140	105–118	137–148	115–129	144–160	125–140
5'6"	5'2"	136–142	108–121	139–151	118–132	146–164	128–144
5'7"	5'3"	138–145	111–124	142–154	121–135	149–168	131–148
5'8"	5'4"	140–148	114–127	145–157	124–138	152–172	134–152
5'9"	5'5"	142–151	117–130	148–160	127–141	155–176	137–156
5'10"	5'6"	144–154	120–133	151–163	130–144	158–180	140–160
5'11"	5'7"	146–157	123–136	154–166	133–147	161–184	143–164
6'0"	5'8"	149–160	126–139	157–170	136–150	164–188	146–167
6'1"	5'9"	152–164	129–142	160–174	139–153	168–192	149–170
6'2"	5'10"	155–168	132–145	164–178	142–156	172–197	152–173

Healthy Fat Intake Per Day[9]

Ideal Weight (in pounds)	Fat Gram Intake (per day)
100	17
105	17.5
110	18
115	19
120	20
125	21
130	21.5
135	22.5
140	23
150	25
160	26
170	28

Note: Men will generally add one more gram of fat per day to their total than women, and people who are very active may add one or two more grams of fat per day to their totals.

Making the Change to the Low-Fat Lifestyle

I do not understand what I do. For what I want to do I do
not do, but what I hate I do.

—ROMANS 7:15

European history tells of two brothers, Edward and Raynald, who were
constantly at war with each other. Raynald, the older of the two, was made
a duke when their father died. But Edward, the younger brother, over-
threw Raynald and took him prisoner.

Why am I telling you this?

Raynald had a weight problem. In fact, he was known among the
population as "Crassus," which means "the Fat." To keep Raynald from
escaping, Edward had a room built around his brother. The windows and
doors of this room were always left open so that Edward could say, "My
brother is not a prisoner. He may leave when he so wills." And this was
true. The only problem was that the windows and doors were smaller than
Raynald was wide, and Edward made sure his older brother was always
well fed. If Raynald wanted to leave his prison, he would have to decline
the regular feasts so he could eventually walk through the open doors.

For ten years Raynald was kept captive, not so much by his brother but by his own appetite. When Edward was eventually killed in battle, Raynald's dukedom was returned to him. Unfortunately, he was now so obese and in such poor health that he died in less than a year.[1]

Can you imagine daily life for Raynald? He could look out the windows and see life going on beyond him. I can just hear him sighing, "If only I could get out of here…," as he saw families strolling by, children at play, and couples walking arm in arm. His life could have had so much fullness, so much richness and joy. Yet there beside him was a table laden with food. Meats, pastries, cheeses. My guess is that, in his misery, he consoled himself with these foods. Perhaps he thought, *Well, if I can't be free, at least I can have the foods I want.* Whatever the case, it's obvious that he didn't have the self-control that would have freed him from his prison and maybe even from the poor health that led to his early death.

It's easy for us to judge Raynald. How could he keep eating when he could have set himself free? Didn't he realize all he was missing? Ten years in prison! Why didn't he simply eat less? Didn't he have any common sense?

Yet as we sit in judgment, we may very well be doing the same things Raynald did. We know that eating better will give us better health, more energy, and greater enjoyment of life. Yet we keep popping Twinkies into our mouths.

Health expert Robert Pritikin puts it this way: "Here is the dark irony of modern life that reveals just how powerful the fattening instinct is. Science has devoted millions of dollars to finding the diet most beneficial to human health. That diet has been discovered, yet no one wants to eat it."[2]

I doubt that much of what I'm sharing with you in these chapters on nutritious eating is new to you. Almost every day we hear about another study describing the benefits of eating vegetables or grains or fruits. Or there's another article stating that obesity is growing at such a fast rate it will soon be considered an epidemic.[3] And then we come across a book about food and politics or food and relationships. The evidence is overwhelming. But, like Raynald, we keep filling up on what we don't need.

Most of us have been like Raynald in another way. We watch others doing things we wish we could do, but we're hampered by our bodies. A dear friend of mine is so overweight that she cannot climb one flight of stairs. She would love to go hiking, swimming, or biking. Yet her body holds her as a prisoner.

This isn't a new problem. In fact, it dates back to that first sin when Eve made a choice to put food in her mouth that didn't belong there. Since then, we've struggled with knowing the right thing to do and actually doing it. We echo the words of the apostle Paul quoted at the beginning of the chapter: "What I want to do I do not do, but what I hate I do." To paraphrase, "I know I shouldn't do this, but I can't seem to stop myself!" It's an ancient problem, and to be honest, the solutions aren't always as simple as they sound.

We all *know* right from wrong. We all *know* that we should eat more wisely. We all *know* that we need to cut back on commitments, nurture our family lives, and spend more time with God. We have all kinds of knowledge, but we still go through life as if we're uninformed and unaware. Why?

We do need knowledge in order to change our lives, but we need a few other things as well. We also need a plan, the ability, support, proper motivation, and God's power. And to possess each of these, we need to take action.

A LITTLE KNOWLEDGE GOES A LONG WAY

Without knowledge, we would have no initial reason to change. Each of us needs to know why changes are called for in our lives. I've already shared with you many reasons to consider making the change to the Low-Fat Lifestyle. If you keep up with the news or are even the most casual of readers, you can't help but read studies or hear of reports that say how good it is to eat fruits, vegetables, and grains—and how damaging it is to consume large quantities of fat and processed foods. We'd be kidding ourselves to say, "I didn't know that wasn't good for me!" We have the knowledge.

As for the action needed in this area, take seriously the knowledge you already have and keep learning more. Believe it when you read that cutting back on fat can help your health. Listen when you hear a report on the effects of too much junk food. Pick up that magazine filled with low-fat recipes, and try some this week. Keep learning as much as you can.

DEVELOP A PLAN OF ACTION

The change to the Low-Fat Lifestyle won't happen by accident. This book will help you plan and make changes in the foods you purchase, prepare, and eat, as well as plan for a fuller life and spiritual growth. As you continue to read, look for practical ideas, places where you're encouraged to keep a journal, or other principles that will help you make change happen.

For example, I know I'll get hungry as I sit at my desk each day, so I keep pretzels and crunchy vegetables on hand. On cold days, I'm sure to have packets of instant oatmeal as a warm and filling snack. By planning for my food needs, I can choose low-fat options instead of heading to the vending machine for a bag of chips or a candy bar. Planning your meals with daily or weekly menus will help you shop for the nutritious foods you'll need. Preparing yourself for meals out, dinner parties, and other events will help you be consistent.

The same kind of planning is also helpful when making day-to-day choices about how to use your time, money, energy, and so on. Having a plan will help you find greater depth in your walk with God. We'll talk about tips and ideas for you to try as we move through the pages of this book. Use these resources to develop a plan so you won't be caught off guard when a challenge comes your way.

RECOGNIZE YOUR ABILITY TO ACHIEVE

Do you have the *ability* to make a positive change in your life? Absolutely! Ability, like knowledge, is something you already possess. When you're handed a plate with several kinds of foods on it, you have the skills necessary to pick out the ones that are best for you. When you're faced with the choice of buying something outside of your budget, you have the ability to choose wisely. When life's demands press in on you from every side, you have the capabilities needed to spend time with God.

Few of us lack the actual physical ability to do what we know is best. However, this is an area where many of us begin to have problems. We start making excuses and placing blame. *Oh, what's the use? I've tried diets and healthy-eating plans before. Nothing works. Besides, my husband won't eat those foods, so I won't bother trying.* When we start thinking like this, we stop seeing that we do have the ability to make changes.

I remember one day when a friend offered me a piece of cheesecake. It was his birthday, and his wife had made the special family recipe for his favorite dessert. I thought, *I shouldn't eat this. I'm not hungry. I've already had plenty.* But my thoughts did not translate into words. In fact, my lips said, "Why, thank you! That cake looks delicious!" My hands, like my lips, ignored my mind and reached out for a slice of cheesecake. And my hands lifted a fork, cut a piece of the cheesecake, and put it into my mouth— right past those badly behaving lips. I ate that one bite and told my friend the cheesecake was scrumptious. It was!

Then my conscience reminded me of my new commitment. I set the cheesecake aside and thought, *There's no law that says I have to finish this. I could make a low-fat cheesecake at home today if I want to eat cheesecake. This one here is nothing but fat, fat, sugar, fat, and more fat.* And then my hands started to obey my mind, and they picked up the cheesecake and tossed it into the trash (but not until my friend had left the room).

I had the ability to choose what was best all along. I just ignored it for a few minutes and let other feelings take over. I thought my friend would be disappointed if I refused his offer of cake, and I let this turn into feelings of guilt. In reality, I could have saved myself a lot of trouble if I'd just said, "No, thanks. I've already eaten." I had the ability to make the right choice, and eventually I used my ability. It just took a while to get started.

Take action by mentally recognizing that you *do* have the ability to make changes. Your actions may not make everyone around you comfortable. Your actions may not be easy. But you *can* make changes. (And take heart, I'll give you a recipe for a delicious low-fat cheesecake later on.)

ENLIST SUPPORTERS

I know exercise is important, but to be honest, I just hate to break a sweat. Walking on a treadmill bores me. Running hurts my back and knees. I'm not good at sports. So it's easy for me to give up on needed exercise. When I make those New Year's resolutions to exercise more, I don't even get started! It's easy for me to break a commitment to myself and say, "I'll try again tomorrow."

Here's the good news: I may stand myself up for an exercise date, but I'd never stand up my sister. If she says, "Let's meet at the lake tomorrow to walk," you can be sure that *I* wouldn't be the thoughtless person who leaves her standing there alone, wondering if she's been abandoned. If I tell her I'll be there, I'll be there! And walking is much more fun if I've got someone to talk to, even if it means I break a sweat. So can you guess my strategy for getting exercise? Yep. Enlist support.

Have you ever considered why so many people trying to overcome addictions join support groups? They need encouragement and account-ability. It's easy to make and break promises in our minds. But when we've made a commitment to someone else, actually said it aloud, maybe even written it down, it's a little harder to back out. Not impossible, of course, but definitely harder.

Support systems give us a place to feel safe and be honest about our needs, desires, and discouragements. Partners can also help us feel loved when we don't feel very lovable, and our need to feel loved is important in breaking habits that have brought us comfort for many years.

Friends, family, and other supporters also can give you the encour-agement you need to stick to your goals. When my friend and I were trav-eling recently, we agreed to eat sensibly and not be tempted by easy-to-find junk food. When one of us said, "No, thanks" when the waiter brought out a tray of fat-laden desserts, it was easier for the other to decline as well.

Find support from people who will be consistent and cheer you on. If your family resists making changes in eating habits, they're not likely to support you. That doesn't mean you can't make the changes; it just means they aren't going to be your cheering section. Instead, find a couple of friends who will join you in your new commitment. Or locate a support group in your community through a health club, local hospital, or other organization. Share your goals for change with these people, and ask them to help you.

Support also comes from within. When you set realistic goals for changing to the Low-Fat Lifestyle, you're supporting yourself. When you read books like this one and learn tips and guidelines for making changes, you're supporting yourself. When you have a positive attitude about adding God's fullness to your life, you're supporting yourself.

Take action today by finding people who will support you. Ask them to encourage you and hold you accountable. See if they'll partner with you. And make sure you give yourself plenty of support through your own actions and attitudes.

DISCOVER THE MAGIC OF MOTIVATION

What is the kick in the pants you need to get you moving? What "carrot" can be dangled in front of you to keep you going forward? What would inspire you to do what is right?

Motivation takes many different forms. Some people are motivated by money, prestige, power, or other rewards. These are largely *external motivators*—things that happen outside of us that prompt us to action. Many of us would not get up in the morning and go to work without the promise of a paycheck. We need the motivation of a reward to keep us employed.

Other people are motivated by the satisfaction of doing a job well, by the desire to help others, or simply because they find joy in their activities. These are *internal motivators*—things that cause us to act because of what's inside us. For example, when our family joined a group of friends for a weekend at a cabin, I soon found myself as the only adult sitting on the floor playing games with all the kids while the other adults chatted over coffee. One parent later thanked me for "taking care of the kids." I laughed because I didn't think of my actions as any kind of childcare. I was having a blast with those kids! My motivation for being with them was simply that I was doing something in which I found great joy.

Both kinds of motivation have their place and neither is right or wrong. However, external motivation doesn't usually lead to lifestyle changes. Once the external motivator is removed, there's no reason to keep moving toward the goal. Consider children who are motivated to learn a Bible verse with the promise of a candy-bar reward. Many churches use this system, and many children do learn Bible verses because of it. But if you stop giving the kids the candy, they'll often stop learning the verses. It's not that the child longs to know God's Word—he or she simply wants the candy enough to do whatever is required. And even though the child may have memorized all the verses, there's no proof the child has made any lifestyle changes as a result of the knowledge.

To make the Low-Fat Lifestyle truly a permanent change and not a temporary "diet," you're going to need internal motivation. Think of it this way: Perhaps you give yourself a small reward for every day you eat properly. Maybe you buy yourself a new outfit or CD each week as a reward for your behavior. But what happens if you're low on funds one week? Do you load up on fat that week because you know you can't reward yourself on Friday?

You actually might want to give yourself occasional external rewards, but if these are your only reason for change, progress is likely to be short-lived. Instead, you need to internally believe that *this change is the best for you and those you love.* You need to take pleasure in eating the delicious foods that will help you enjoy good health. Remember, this is life to the fullest! If you truly believe that, then you won't need payment or prestige to keep you on track. The reward for this lifestyle change is that you will enjoy better health, have more energy, and be better equipped physically to make the most of your relationships with family, friends, and God.

Take action by considering what things motivate you in other areas of life. Do you do things for external rewards or for internal satisfaction? What might help you adjust your attitude in this area? Where would external motivators be helpful to you, and where will they quickly become meaningless? Focus on the internal joy you'll discover in this new lifestyle.

PLUG IN TO GOD'S POWER

When the apostle Paul was writing to the Roman believers, he expressed his frustration at his own actions. He tended to do what he knew was wrong and to not do what he knew was right. To solve this problem, Paul didn't say, "Just do it!" Instead, he recognized that sin is a strong enemy and that God's power was needed for him to do what was right. Listen as he grappled with this issue:

> For I have the desire to do what is good, but I cannot carry it out.
> For what I do is not the good I want to do; no, the evil I do not want
> to do—this I keep on doing. Now if I do what I do not want to do,
> it is no longer I who do it, but it is sin living in me that does it.
> So I find this law at work: When I want to do good, evil is right

there with me. For in my inner being I delight in God's law; but I see another law at work in the members of my body, waging war against the law of my mind and making me a prisoner of the law of sin at work within my members. What a wretched man I am! Who will rescue me from this body of death? Thanks be to God—through Jesus Christ our Lord! (Romans 7:18-25)

Paul's comments remind me again of Raynald and his imprisonment. Without self-control, the portly brother was a prisoner, essentially locked in his cell. Likewise, without God, we are prisoners to sin—locked into behaviors we know are wrong.

For many of us, poor habits go deeper than our own abilities, deeper than our knowledge, and they are just as much a prison as the walls that held Raynald. One researcher says, "We are most successful when we also address the emotional and spiritual dimensions that most influence what we choose to do or not do." This doctor asked his patients why, even with all the knowledge they had, they still made poor choices in eating and lifestyle. Their most frequent response: pain. People overate to cope with their emotional and spiritual pain.[4]

Gary Smalley, best known for his books and teachings on interpersonal relationships, has gone through his own battle with this issue as it relates to eating. As he gained weight through poor eating habits, he began to despair at his lack of self-control. He shares how he came to rely on God's power:

I knew that I was out of options other than this last-ditch attempt: to give my struggle to God and seek his best for my life, through his strength alone.

So I got on my knees and cried out to God. I patterned my cry after the passage in Psalms, "Call upon me in the day of trouble; I will deliver you, and you will honor me."

Still on my knees, I admitted that I could not control my eating, that I had tried, and that the task was beyond me. My own abilities were not sufficient. I came to God and said, "I can't seem to do this on my own. It's not going to happen through my own efforts."

After a time of crying out to God, Smalley relates, "He began to make even clearer the definition of his strength in my life. God alone can give us the power to live life fully. That's really it in a few words."[5]

Paul recognized it. Gary Smalley recognized it. And you and I must recognize it as well. All our human knowledge, abilities, support, and motivation can fail us. Only God will not. Only he has the power to change our lives. Our own attempts are sure to fail unless we turn to God for strength.

Later we will more fully address our relationship with God and how it affects every area of our lives, but take action now by asking God to give you his strength, power, and grace to make the changes necessary for low-fat living. Approach God often, asking for his help. He will give it!

To encourage you further, consider these promises from God's Word:

But we have this treasure in jars of clay to show that this all-surpassing power is from God and not from us. (2 Corinthians 4:7)

God is able to make all grace abound to you, so that in all things at all times, having all that you need, you will abound in every good work. (2 Corinthians 9:8)

Now to him who is able to do immeasurably more than all we ask
or imagine, according to his power that is at work within us, to
him be glory in the church and in Christ Jesus throughout all generations, for ever and ever! (Ephesians 3:20-21)

Therefore, prepare your minds for action; be self-controlled; set
your hope fully on the grace to be given you when Jesus Christ is
revealed. As obedient children, do not conform to the evil desires
you had when you lived in ignorance. But just as he who called
you is holy, so be holy in all you do; for it is written: "Be holy,
because I am holy." (1 Peter 1:13-16)

I encourage you to copy one or more of these verses onto cards and
put them around your home, your office, and in your car—wherever
you'll see them. Think on them often, and look to God for your strength
as you choose the Low-Fat Lifestyle. Rely on the One who can do "immeasurably more than all we ask or imagine."

THREE

The Low-Fat Kitchen

How priceless is your unfailing love! Both high and low among men find refuge in the shadow of your wings. They feast on the abundance of your house; you give them drink from your river of delights.

—PSALM 36:7-8

I once interviewed the author of a nutrition cookbook. The pictures of the prepared dishes looked lovely, but the ingredients made me cringe. First, I had no idea where I would purchase all the exotic ingredients. Second, the names of the ingredients sounded awful. I couldn't figure out how the author or the photographer or the food stylist had turned things that sounded like puréed grass and bark (imported from Spain, of course) into an attractive side dish.

The author assured me the food tasted great and that if I started eating these nutritious items, I'd never turn back to a chocolate bar again. Believe me when I say I had a chocolate bar in my mouth within five minutes of the interview. There was no way I was going to eat as she did.

This author and I were not at entirely opposite ends of the spectrum. After all, my family did eat vegetables occasionally, and we didn't have dessert with breakfast (at least not every day). But there were plenty of differences in our attitudes toward food.

In his book *Food and Love,* Gary Smalley tells about a time he was preparing to use his chainsaw. In a hurry, he accidentally poured oil into the gasoline tank and gasoline into the oil reservoir. His chainsaw didn't work, and it took him a while to figure out what he'd done wrong. When it was over, he came up with the simple truth that applies to humans: We not only need fuel, but we need the *right* fuel.[1]

Just because our bodies need food—nutritious food—doesn't mean we have to eat tasteless and difficult-to-prepare meals. It doesn't mean our food has to taste like puréed grass and bark. And it doesn't mean we have to spend every Saturday chasing down obscure ingredients. We can eat delicious foods that are good for us and easy to prepare.

PONDERING THE FOOD PYRAMID

Let's take stock of your kitchen right now and see what should and shouldn't be there. As a guide, we'll use a helpful chart created by the U.S. Department of Agriculture: the Food Guide Pyramid. Following this guide will give us an idea of how much food we can eat each day (and believe me, it allows for plenty of food).

We'll also refer to the "Nutrition Facts" information that's legally required on all packaged food. This chart, which is usually found on the side of a box or can, tells how much of the product constitutes one serving and how many calories, grams of fat, and vitamins are in that serving.

As we move up the Food Guide Pyramid, you might notice that what you normally eat is out of proportion with the recommendations. Many of us think of meat as the main portion of our meal while bread, fruits, and vegetables serve as side dishes. Yet the food pyramid clearly shows us that it should be the other way around. As we explore how to get the most from our foods, keep in mind that you may need to adjust your thinking on what makes a healthy, nutritious meal.

The Food Guide Pyramid

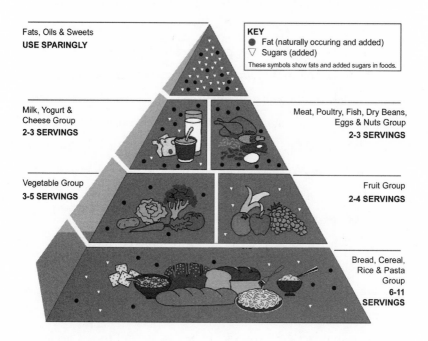

(Source: U.S. Department of Agriculture and U.S. Department of Human Services)

Bread, Cereal, Rice, and Pasta: 6–11 Daily Servings

Let's start at the bottom of the Food Guide Pyramid and work our way to the top. The base of the pyramid forms the foundation for our eating. This is where many diets lose people because they recommend avoiding breads, rice, and pasta. Yet these foods give us a full feeling and can offer many nutrients our bodies need. And we can have a lot of them too. Even with the minimum allowance of six servings, I could have a bowl of cereal for breakfast, half a bagel for a midmorning snack, a sandwich for lunch, a roll with dinner, and a bowl of popcorn later in the evening. That's a lot of food—and it's only from one group!

Grains provide our bodies with vitamins and minerals as well as fiber. Some grains also provide protein. However, the more grains are processed, the more nutrients they lose. Since we want all the good stuff we can get, look for products that use whole grains and have the fewest additives.

With all foods in this group, be sure you check the serving size. For example, a large muffin you grab from the vending machine at work may actually be so large that it counts as two or more servings. Read the label on the side of a package to see how much of the product you should eat to have one serving. In general, one slice of bread is a serving, one cup of packaged cereal (such as cornflakes) is a serving, and one-half cup of rice, pasta, or cooked cereal (such as oatmeal) is a serving.

Bread. When you shop for bread at the grocery store, you'll find a variety of choices labeled "low-fat." Unfortunately, many of these are flimsy bits of bread with no substance. In fact, some are similar in content to regular bread and have simply been cut into thinner slices so that the fat-per-serving is less. Still, you should be able to find breads made with whole grains that don't have a lot of added oil. Sourdough bread is usually low in fat and is dense enough to be filling (and to not fall apart when you add a few slices of tomato and cucumber between two pieces).

Our family has found the best breads at a bakery several miles from our home. We purchase a few loaves at a time and store them in the freezer. This bakery uses freshly ground wheat and other grains, honey instead of sugar and oil, and doesn't add unwanted preservatives. Look around your neighborhood, and talk to bakery employees. Good bread is out there.

You may also choose to make your own bread. There's nothing like the aroma of homemade bread! Bread machines are popular, or you can stick with the old-fashioned method and knead your bread by hand. Either way, look for recipes and mixes that use little or no oil so you can enjoy your bread without consuming unwanted fats. (In chapter 5, I've included an easy recipe that can be used for loaves of bread or dinner rolls.)

Cereal. I'm not a big fan of cold cereal—too many memories of soggy Cheerios as a child, I guess. But the rest of my family loves cereal any time of day. My son likes to take a bowl of cereal to school and pour his little carton of milk over it for his lunch. And cereal is a regular nighttime snack for my husband.

Look for cereals that are high in fiber and low in sugar and fat. Be careful about some of the "health food" cereals, such as granola, as these are often baked in oils and can be very fatty. In fact, one box I saw at the supermarket recently revealed that one-half cup of a certain brand of granola had 10 grams of fat. That's terrible! We should be able to eat hearty grains without someone pouring fat on top of them. Some companies do make these cereals without the added fat, so read labels carefully.

Hot cereals are generally low in fat and high in fiber and nutrients. They also tend to be filling and satisfying. I keep a few packets of instant oatmeal at my desk. If I get hungry for something warm, I add a little water in my mug, zap it in the microwave, and have a satisfying snack in minutes.

Rice and Pasta. Rice and pasta also provide nutrients we need, and they give a satisfying feeling of being full. Most people don't like these foods plain, so rice and pasta are often cooked with oils or covered with gravies or sauces. There are many ways to prepare great-tasting rice and pasta without all the added fat; for example, try preparing them in fat-free chicken or vegetable broth. (See chapter 5 for recipes that include these foods.)

Other Grains. This category includes tortillas, dinner rolls, muffins, corn bread, and more. The list of foods made with grains goes on and on. As you eat your six to eleven servings of these foods each day, remember to read labels to make sure you're getting enough nutrients and not exceeding the serving size. Also be on the lookout for fat hidden in some of these products. For example, purchased muffins are usually very high in fat, as are croissants and corn chips.

When I found tasty-looking "low-fat" tortilla chips at my grocery store, I turned the bag over to see how much fat was in one serving. Only 1 gram per serving. But then I looked to see how big a serving was: eight chips. *Eight chips?* How do you fill up on eight? Nearby was another bag of tortilla chips that also claimed to be low in fat. These chips also had only 1 gram of fat per serving, but this time the serving was eighteen chips. That's more like it! Reading labels allowed me to eat enough chips to feel like I'd actually had a snack, without adding unwanted grams of fat.

What to Keep, What to Toss. Get rid of the fatty croissants, corn chips, and granolas. If you feel guilty throwing away food, use it to fill your bird feeder. Restock your shelves with hearty breads, baked chips, and lower-fat cereals. Stock up on oatmeal, rice, and pasta. You'll be eating a lot of these foods!

Vegetables: 3–5 Daily Servings; Fruit: 2–4 Daily Servings

Are you a fan of *VeggieTales,* the videos and books that feature characters right out of your produce section? Did you know that Bob the Tomato and Larry the Cucumber aren't really veggies at all? They're fruits! Telling fruits and vegetables apart has to do with where the seeds are (and other biology stuff that gets confusing), so since fruits and vegetables are often so hard to tell apart, let's talk about them all at once.

When our son was young, he went grocery shopping with me every week. From a child's point of view, the grocery store has got to be a marvelous place. Brightly colored cartons, cartoon-character faces popping off of every container, promises of toys inside boxes. So much to look at and so much to buy! Tony, like many children, began to develop a habit of asking for just about everything at the grocery store.

"Can we buy that cereal? Can I have that candy? I want some of those! Let's buy that!"

I felt like the bad guy saying no all the time. But I had to. First of all, I simply couldn't afford to buy everything Tony wanted. And second, a lot of the things he asked for were junk. I wanted Tony to love good foods, not junk food.

One day, I hit upon an idea that changed everything. As we rounded the corner to the produce section of the grocery store, I spread my arms to the vast array of colorful fruits and vegetables. Then I said, "Tony, you can choose *anything* you want from this area. Every week you can choose whatever you want and as much as you want from this area, and I'll buy it."

Tony, who was about four years old at the time, smiled his most endearing smile. He jumped off the end of the cart and began exploring. During the following weeks and months, he chose a wide variety of foods he'd previously turned his nose up at, such as Brussels sprouts and asparagus. He got our whole family to try foods I'd never even heard of—things like carambola and Bosc pears. We've eaten eggplant, an array of squashes, oranges from other countries, apples of all colors, kumquats, snow peas, plantains, and persimmons. I've had to hunt down store employees who could tell us the names of these foods and how to eat or prepare them. It was an adventure.

The amazing thing about fruits and vegetables is how good they are for you. I'm always finding studies showing how eating more broccoli, or more leafy vegetables, or more apples, or more *anything* from this food group has been found to lengthen life, boost energy, lower the chances of getting cancer, and on and on. This stuff is great for you!

Fruits and vegetables do have trace amounts of fat in them, but it's often so low it's not worth counting. For example, one cup of diced cantaloupe has .2 grams of fat. A cup of raw carrots has .1 grams of fat. So you could eat cup after cup of these and still not eat a full gram of fat. The exceptions are avocados and olives. Putting one tablespoon of avocado on a sandwich adds about 2.5 grams of fat. A serving of ten olives has between 5 and 7 grams of fat, depending on the type and size of olive.

Begin experimenting with fruits and vegetables. Try something you've never had before. Keep bowls of fruit on your counter. Grate or chop vegetables into your casseroles. Choose 100 percent fruit or vegetable juices instead of soft drinks. Carry bags of snow peas, sliced peppers, and cherry tomatoes along to the office. Veggies are great snacks since they're so low in calories, are nearly fat-free, and are full of nutrients.

Chapter 5 has only a few recipes for fruits and vegetables. That's because these foods are so good they don't need much preparation or improvement. Steam vegetables or serve them raw. Offer fruit as a salad or a dessert. Raid your spice cabinet and experiment with different seasonings. Tony used to call fruit "God's candy," and it's true! These foods are good just as they are.

What to Keep, What to Toss. French fries and onion rings don't count as low-fat vegetables. Skip those and stock your kitchen with fresh and frozen fruits and vegetables. The more the better! Keep them handy and ready to eat. Let these become your new snack foods. Store a few bags of dried fruits in the cabinet—they're so sweet and tasty! Every time you prepare a meal, steam a pan of vegetables or cut slices of fruit and leave them on the table for everyone to enjoy.

Milk, Yogurt, and Cheese: 2–3 Daily Servings

Moving up the pyramid, we find milk, yogurt, and cheese, often referred to as the dairy group. From these we get protein, vitamins, calcium, and other important nutrients. Also, in the form of sauces and toppings, these items add flavor to many of the other foods we like. However, as these foods are also animal products, they tend to be high in fat. The good news is that we don't have to completely eliminate these foods from our plates. We just need to take extra care in which of these we buy and how we use them.

The milk, yogurt, and cheese group is not a difficult one to adapt for the Low-Fat Lifestyle. Almost every dairy product is available without fat. I realize that if you're used to drinking whole milk, skim milk tastes pretty watery. In that case, make a gradual change. Switch to 2 percent for one or two weeks, then move to 1 percent for another week or two. When you make the final step to skim milk, the change will not be as drastic. Skim milk still has all the calcium and other nutrients you gain from whole milk, but without the fat you don't need.

Fat-free yogurt, sour cream, coffee creamer, cottage cheese, and most other dairy products taste almost the same as their high-fat counterparts. As with milk, if the change in taste seems too drastic for you, try the low-fat variety first, and when you're accustomed to that, move to the fat-free version.

Cheeses that are completely fat free are difficult to find. If none are available in your area, use low-fat cheeses, which are readily available. However, be sure you measure cheese when you use it. This is one food on which it's easy to overindulge. What seems like just a sprinkling to you might actually be several servings. Read the labels and measure cheese when you add it to sandwiches and other recipes. To help you begin reducing the amount of cheese in your diet, try using a stronger-flavored cheese but in smaller amounts. You'll still get a lot of flavor but much less fat.

If you're cooking for people besides yourself, you may have to make some concessions in this area. It was easy for our family to begin drinking skim milk and eating fat-free yogurt and sour cream. My son, however, does not care for fat-free cream cheese, and I don't like fat-free mozzarella. In these cases, we eat less of the low-fat varieties. If you choose to go for the added flavor of a higher-fat food, remember to figure the added grams of fat into your daily allowance.

What to Keep, What to Toss. This is an easy one. Toss those cartons of high-fat dairy products, and replace them with their low-fat and no-fat equivalents.

Meat, Poultry, Fish, Dry Beans, Eggs, and Nuts: 2–3 Daily Servings

Right next to the dairy foods on the pyramid we find meat, poultry, fish, dry beans, eggs, and nuts. Like dairy foods, these also provide protein and other nutrients. Unfortunately, many foods in this group also contain a lot of fat.

As I mentioned earlier, we generally think of meat as the main portion of our meal and relegate the other foods to the role of side dishes. The pyramid turns this around. If we eat only the recommended two to three servings from the meat, poultry, fish, dry beans, eggs, and nuts group, it's clear that we need to consider bread, fruits, and vegetables as our main courses with just a small amount of meat, eggs, or nuts on the side.

Meat, Poultry, Fish, and Eggs. Our doctor has recommended that we not eat any foods from this group, and several books we've read on healthful eating confirm this recommendation. Even though meat, poultry, fish, and eggs do provide protein, they also contain fat, cholesterol, and chemicals that can be harmful to our bodies. These animal products don't supply any fiber, and they are often cooked in oils.

Other experts feel there should be a more balanced approach to eating, one more in line with the Food Guide Pyramid, which allows two or three servings of foods from this group each day.

Our family has found a middle ground. We have chosen not to eat any red meat, pork, or egg yolks (where all the fat is). We do eat small portions of skinless white meat from chicken and turkey, and egg whites (which have a lot of protein but only trace amounts of fat). Those of us who like fish eat it occasionally, but since it's not a family favorite, it has not been hard to eliminate. This is an area about which you'll have to reach your own conclusions. It is a challenge to eliminate a food group entirely, but it's not impossible if you feel strongly about it.

When you eat poultry, eat only the white meat, and always remove the skin before cooking. Leaving the skin on adds several grams of fat.

If you crave red meats but want to avoid the fat, try ostrich! We had this for the first time when we were eating at a restaurant. As we looked over the menu, we saw many exotic dishes and didn't know which would be lowest in fat. After talking to the waiter, Mike tried a dish with ostrich meat. It looks and tastes like red meat but has even less fat than chicken or turkey breast. We've found an exotic-meats butcher nearby who sells ground ostrich and ostrich steaks. If you want to try this meat, ask your butcher where to find it, or purchase it online. It can be expensive, so you might want to save it for special occasions.

When you do eat meat, choose very lean cuts and try to limit yourself to one serving per day. One serving of lean meat, poultry, or fish is two to three ounces—about the size of a deck of cards. That's not much, and it's certainly less than the huge portions we may be accustomed to serving ourselves.

Meats also should be prepared without added fats. Grilled or baked meats can still be tender and flavorful without the added fat that frying requires. Many marinades can be made or purchased without oil, and they also add a variety of flavors to meats. As our desire is to get the most from our foods, I've included recipes in chapter 5 that allow you to enjoy small amounts of meats while filling yourself with grains, fruits, and vegetables.

When eating eggs, use two egg whites in place of one whole egg. You may also purchase egg substitutes in small cartons. Simply measure the amount given on the product (usually one-quarter to one-third of a cup), and add this to your recipe. Egg substitutes can also be used for omelets and scrambled eggs, but they can be expensive. It's actually cheaper to buy regular eggs and throw away unused yolks (just crack the egg into your hand, and let the white seep through your fingers). Yes, this is wasting food, but it also eliminates something your body doesn't need.

Dry Beans and Nuts. These are the plant alternatives to the other foods in this category. When beans are combined with a grain or a dairy product, they form a complete protein; thus meats are not required to supply the protein we need for a healthy diet. A plate of black beans and rice flavored with onions, peppers, and tomatoes is a low-fat meal that's filling and protein-rich.

Nuts have protein as well, and since they're plant-based, the fat in them is not as harmful to your body as animal fat. But the fat content of nuts *is* high. A handful of large cashews (approximately fourteen) has almost 13 grams of fat; one tablespoon of chopped pecans has 5 grams of fat; and one tablespoon of chopped peanuts has 4.5 grams of fat. Almonds have less fat (just under 4 grams per tablespoon) and are usually not cooked in additional oil, so they're a better choice if you do eat nuts.

One problem many people have with nuts is that they're easy to snack on and hard to stop eating. It may be easier for you to leave them out of your diet completely or use them sparingly as a garnish or for some added flavor and crunch in a vegetable dish or salad.

What to Keep, What to Toss. Before you shop, determine what kinds of meat you're going to select. Then either walk past the butcher section of the grocery store or at least walk past the fatty meats and choose the leanest ones possible. Ask for skinless chicken breast, ground turkey made with only white meat, and the fish with the lowest fat. Many products that are commonly made with pork are now available made from turkey— turkey bacon, turkey pepperoni, turkey sausage, and more. Be sure to read the labels and serve appropriate portions, and you'll find you can still have lots of flavor without all the fat.

Explore the options available with soy burgers or other "burgers" made with vegetables and soy. Buy a small amount, and try these as meat substitutes. If you like them, choose them over meat whenever possible.

Use a food scale to see how much meat you're serving yourself and your family. Remember, meat is a side dish and portions should be small. Grab a few low-fat frozen meals, and store them in the freezer for occasional quick meals. These are already packaged in portion-controlled servings and are quick to prepare.

Fats, Oils, and Sweets: Use Sparingly

Finally, we reach the tiny area at the top of the pyramid. This little section shows us that fats, oils, and sweets should be the smallest amount of food that we eat. It's interesting to note that there's no recommended serving on this portion of the chart. The chart shows symbols to indicate fat and sugar, and you may have noticed that these symbols also appear throughout the other areas, as sugars and fats are found in many foods.

Many people get worried about this section of the pyramid. After all, we like butter on our bread and Ranch dressing on our salads. Don't worry. I like to eat food that tastes great too, and I have found many ways to increase flavor while decreasing fat. Keep reading, and you'll find you can do it too!

In your kitchen, you'll find oil in various forms. It's a liquid in bottles of vegetable oil, olive oil, sunflower oil, and so on. It's a solid in the form of butter, margarine, and shortening or lard. Despite its varied form, it's all fat. Read the label on the side of the container, and see how much fat is in a tablespoon of each product. Depending on what you're looking at, you'll see a tablespoon of oil has between 11 and 14 grams of fat per tablespoon. Yikes! Let's say that our fictional friend Jennie has decided to allot herself 10 percent of her calories from fat (20 grams of fat a day). So if she divides one tablespoon of butter between two pieces of toast for breakfast, she has only 6 grams of fat left for the whole day.

Before our family made the switch to the Low-Fat Lifestyle, I purchased at least one pound of butter or margarine each week—plus additional bottles of oil and tubs of shortening. Now that we've changed our lifestyle, I purchase about two pounds of butter and one small bottle of olive oil per *year!* I do have these on hand for a few recipes that use a tablespoon of butter or oil, or for when company comes for dinner. (Although

I prepare low-fat meals, I don't want to force my choices on guests. And I do let them put butter on their dinner roll!)

Other sources of almost pure oil you'll find in your kitchen are mayonnaise and salad dressings. Most brands of mayonnaise have about 11 grams of fat per tablespoon—about the amount you'd put on a sandwich. And salad dressings are often just as bad. Many people think they're eating healthy by choosing a salad instead of a burger and fries. Sure, the salad is filled with many wonderful vegetables, but it might be coated with almost pure oil. It's possible to consume more fat in a salad than you would in a burger and fries.

Oils and fats hide in many foods, and we want to uncover those hidden sources. But we pour oil right on many foods without even thinking twice. You know how easy it is to slather butter or margarine on vegetables and breads. What about all the oil in which we fry so many of our foods? How much oil do you add to the batter when you're baking? How much mayonnaise do you add to a potato salad? When you start adding up those fat grams, you quickly realize how easy it is to exceed your limit.

SEARCHING FOR LOW-FAT SOLUTIONS

With so many tantalizing dishes loaded with high-fat oils, how can we be expected to maintain the Low-Fat Lifestyle? Don't despair. There are many alternatives to the kinds of oils we want to avoid.

If you absolutely must use oil, choose olive oil—but use it sparingly. Studies show that this natural fat has some health benefits, such as increasing the good cholesterol in your blood. However, all oils are high in fat and as there are alternatives in most cases, choose the low-fat and fat-free options whenever you can.

Baking

I love to bake, and I love to eat baked goods. I was relieved to learn that in many recipes for baked goods—such as brownies, cakes, and cookies—you can substitute a variety of things for oil. Look on the aisle where shortening and baking goods are sold at your grocery store: You'll find oil and shortening replacements there. One I use often is Lighter Bake, which consists mostly of puréed prunes. I know, it sounds awful, but it really does make foods moist without adding oil. If the thought of using prunes in your brownies doesn't make you happy, you can use applesauce instead and get a similar result. If you use puréed prunes or applesauce, remember that you do *not* use the same amount as you would with oil. Instead, you use half the amount of the puréed fruit to replace the oil.

There are other brands of oil replacements available at the grocery store, some of which are used in amounts equivalent to oil. You'll want to read the labels and instructions on these products so your baked goods don't turn out too moist or too dry.

Another food that works well as an oil substitute in many baked goods is fat-free sour cream. Try this when making pancakes, coffee cakes, and sweet breads. Use the same amount of fat-free sour cream as you would oil.

Frying

What about when a recipe calls for vegetables to be sautéed or cooked in oil until tender? In this case, you can skip the oil completely and use white wine or fat-free chicken broth to soften onions, green peppers, mushrooms, or other foods. You can even simmer foods in water, but the flavor is not as good. No matter which liquid you choose, simply pour about one-half cup into your frying pan, and add the vegetables you want sautéed. Add more liquid as needed, and cook until the food is tender.

When it comes to foods like fried chicken, you will have to use a tiny bit of oil. But, to be honest, you're going to have to give up most deep-fried foods. There simply isn't a way to immerse a piece of food into a vat of hot oil and not have the food absorb quite a bit of the oil. (You'll find a low-fat recipe for "fried" chicken in chapter 5.) You can also experiment with other ways to get the fried flavor without actually soaking up all the oil. For example, you might try lightly coating foods with cooking spray and then baking them. You'll often get a crispy food with much less fat.

Butter and Margarine

Many people like breads with melted butter dripping off the sides. Have you ever tasted bread without butter? If you buy or make good quality bread, you'll find it tastes great without all the extra fat on top. The bakery where I shop makes delicious fat-free bread, which doesn't need additional flavor from butter.

My family does not share my fondness for plain bread, so we've experimented with different brands of "light" and low-fat butter-flavored sprays and spreads. Some of these are tasty. Use them sparingly for added flavor, and look for brands that use natural ingredients. Remember that foods with less than .5 grams of fat per serving may be labeled fat-free. So if you use more than one serving, you will be getting fat from this "fat-free" product. For example, some margarine sprays are fat-free if you use less than three squirts. If you pump the bottle ten or twenty times, you'll be adding several grams of fat to your bread.

This is also a time to enjoy the flavors of fruit jams and preserves or honey. None of these have fat, and they add wonderful flavor to bread. Try the butter and margarine substitutes on vegetables as well. Again, I prefer my vegetables without extra flavorings. I love the flavors God gave them and don't think veggies need any help from me. But if you're used to buttered vegetables, try a substitute. Your grocery store has dry butter-flavored crystals and powders in the aisle where spices are sold.

Salad Dressing

Toss the mayonnaise that's in your fridge, and purchase a jar of the fat-free variety. It works just as well in recipes, and you won't find much difference in flavor on sandwiches.

Salad dressing is one area where many of the fat-free equivalents have not been able to match the taste of the fat-laden ones. There are many bottled fat-free dressings, and if you find the flavor acceptable, choose from these. Usually, the Italian dressings and ones with similar flavors taste great. But the Ranch and other creamy varieties often are lacking. If you can't stand the taste, try one of the low-fat varieties, which have excellent flavor and are still low in fat.

I encourage you to experiment with new ways to eat salad. Try leaving off the dressing and using a splash of red wine vinegar and a dash of black pepper instead. Or spritz fresh lemon juice over your greens. Most of us don't like our greens dry, so find ways to add a little moisture and flavor that don't add in the fat.

Other Toppings

As with salads, we often add fatty toppings to our foods, not just for flavor but also for moisture. A baked potato doesn't really need a glob of sour cream on top. Instead, use a bit of fat-free sour cream and skim milk. The milk will add moisture so the potato won't be so dry. Gravies can be made or purchased with little or no fat, as can many other sauces. Experiment with recipes and try new products you'll find at the grocery store.

What to Keep, What to Toss

Toss the oils, margarines, butters, mayonnaise, and so on. Replace them with low-fat and fat-free alternatives. Keep one small bottle of olive oil for occasional use, and begin trying other flavorful options on your foods. Try a few new flavors of jam or jelly. Keep the single-serving sizes of applesauce in the cabinet to use when baking. Purchase new spices to add flavor to foods without adding fat.

PACKAGED SNACKS AND DESSERTS

Because so many people are realizing the benefits of consuming less fat, food companies are providing more and more low-fat options. You'll find many fat-free products at your grocery store. Keep in mind, however, that you can defeat your low-fat eating plan by overindulging in foods such as fat-free cookies and chips. Focus on the plant-based foods on the Food Guide Pyramid as your primary foods. Load your plate with grains, fruits, and vegetables, and let one fat-free brownie be the treat to satisfy your sweet tooth. Don't do it the other way, with a plate of fat-free brownies and a carrot for dessert—you'll miss out on all the nutrition and fullness of the Low-Fat Lifestyle.

What to Keep, What to Toss

Keep low-fat and fat-free snacks on hand, but not too many. If you're like most people, whatever is handiest to grab when you're hungry is what goes into your mouth. Make sure fruits and vegetables are the easiest items to grab, and set aside sweet treats for desserts. Make a rule in your house that sweets are not snacks.

WHAT NEXT?

Look through your kitchen. Open the cabinets, the refrigerator, and the freezer. Read the labels on the foods you've got. Then begin tossing out the foods that are high in fat. You need to make room in your kitchen for all the delicious low-fat foods that are going to start filling your home. Here are a few quick tips on filling those shelves:

- While grocery shopping, read the labels as you go. It will take extra time for the first few weeks, so don't shop when you're feeling rushed. After a few weeks, you'll quickly recognize foods that are low in fat and high in taste and nutrition.

- Target fresh foods as much as possible. Generally, the more processed foods are, the more things have been added that your body doesn't need. But frozen fruits and vegetables are handy to keep in your kitchen since you can always add them to a meal or have them for a snack.

- Although frozen meals are not the most healthful choice, they can come in handy if you're not much of a cook, or if you rely on frozen foods for lunches or quick meals. You'll find a variety of frozen meals that are low in fat and still offer an ample portion of food. These meals usually are heavy on vegetables and rice or pasta and have just enough meat to add flavor. Store a few of these in the freezer so you can have a low-fat meal available the next time you're in a hurry.

- Pretzels, popcorn or puffed-rice cakes, low-fat or fat-free crackers, and baked chips make crunchy snacks that don't cause you any guilt. Keep these on hand for the times you need a nibble. Try keeping some in your desk or car so that when hunger strikes, you can snack healthfully instead of stopping for a carton of fries or hitting the vending machines.
- Purchase an inexpensive scale to weigh foods. The kind used to weigh postage in your home works fine, or check cooking supply shops. These will help you figure out portions measured in ounces, such as meats and foods you prepare at home.

As you restock your kitchen with foods that are full of goodness, be prepared to be well-fed and to leave the table feeling satisfied. That's what God has in store for you!

Eating Out the Low-Fat Way (and Loving It!)

So whether you eat or drink or whatever you do, do it all
for the glory of God.

—1 CORINTHIANS 10:31

No time to cook? Consider these facts about Americans and their love
for eating out:

- Americans generally eat more than four meals a week away from
  home.[1]
- In 2001, Americans spent more than $110 billion on fast
  food.[2]
- Forty-four percent of the money Americans spend on food is
  spent on food eaten outside the home.[3]
- One-fourth of American adults eat fast food each day.[4]
- The average American eats three hamburgers and four orders of
  French fries each week.[5]
- Each American eats about twenty-eight pounds of French fries
  each year.[6]

- The food industry spends $10 billion a year on direct media advertising, compared to approximately $2 million that's spent encouraging the public to eat fruits and vegetables.[7]
- An additional $20 billion is spent each year on indirect marketing for food industry products.[8]

The food industry, especially fast-food and chain restaurants, spends enormous amounts of money on marketing and advertising. Sure, we see the heartwarming or humorous commercials on television, and we flip past the advertisements in our favorite magazines. But what about the backpacks, lunchboxes, gym scoreboards, T-shirts, water bottles, and so on that feature logos and characters from food-related businesses? This indirect marketing is always around us, urging us to not only eat at a certain location but also to eat, eat, eat. Isn't it funny to think that people are selling us the idea of eating? They want us to eat more so they can make more money.

There's truly nothing wrong with eating out. Despite the discouraging information about how much money we spend and how much fat we consume while dining out, there is good news: You *can* eat out and find foods that are low in fat and high in nutrition. You may have to look a little harder, but they're there!

This chapter will help you navigate your way through a variety of restaurants. There's no need to swear off eating out altogether—just a need to look for the healthful foods and fill up on them.

When Mike and I were first married, eating out was an extravagance. Even stopping for fast food was rare since we were poor college students subsisting mostly on macaroni and cheese. As the years went by and we had more disposable income, it became easier to stop for fast food or go out with friends. When Tony was young, we established a habit of going out for fast food each Sunday after church—a tradition we continue to this day.

But when Mike became sick, our fast-food and restaurant habits changed considerably. Initially, it was simply too much trouble to figure out how much fat he was going to be served when eating away from our home. In fact, even eating at friends' homes wasn't easy (and we'll talk about that later). After quite a bit of research, we discovered which low-fat foods are served at most restaurants and how to select and order these foods. Mike began venturing out and eating low-fat foods. Tony and I, however, kept on eating burgers and fries as before.

As I shared earlier, the more I saw Mike benefit from the Low-Fat Lifestyle and the more I learned about the harmful effects of many of the foods I was eating, I, too, began to choose more healthful foods. Now the thought of eating a hamburger covered with cheese, mayonnaise, bacon, and who knows what else makes my stomach turn. I cringe just looking at these foods on television commercials. But I still enjoy dining out, and here's how you can too.

STRATEGY #1: BECOME SERVING-SIZE SAVVY

Let's start with the issue of portion control. Virtually every fast-food restaurant offers the option to upsize, supersize, megasize, or otherwise enlarge your order. Even their "value meals"—where you pay a slightly lower price for a package including a sandwich, onion rings or fries, and a beverage—are means to get you to order and eat more food.

In restaurants, portion sizes have gotten wildly out of control. One report showed that restaurants now serve portions that are "seven times the size recommended by government nutrition experts."[9] I recently dined in a restaurant and was served a bowl of pasta that easily would have fed three people. Another time I told the waiter I'd just have the salad, thinking I'd be brought a bowl about the size of a cereal bowl. Instead, he brought out a bowl of salad that my whole family wouldn't have finished in three days. We've become so accustomed to seeing huge plates piled with food that we're disappointed when we get "only" what we need.

Here are some tips for becoming portion-size wise. Remember that as long as you're eating nutritious, low-fat foods, you can eat until you're full. But there's no need to stuff yourself until you have to let your belt out a notch. First, keep in mind how big a true serving is. When we're eating out, it's tricky to estimate the amount of food on our plates, so here are some practical guidelines:

- Half a cup of any food (rice, pasta, hot cereal, fruit, vegetable) is about the size of a woman's fist.
- One serving of meat is two to three ounces, approximately the size of a deck of cards.
- One serving of bread is the equivalent of one slice of sandwich bread.
- One ounce of cheese is about four chunks the size of dice.

As you measure and weigh foods in your home, pay attention to the size of the portions. This will help you become familiar with what you should be eating at a restaurant. One person I heard about even drew sketches of how big a piece of chicken, a scoop of rice, or a bowl of fruit should be. She kept these handy and gave them a quick glance when dining out to be sure she was consuming reasonable portions.

When you're served a gigantic portion, immediately cut the meal in half or thirds and determine how much you'll eat and how much you'll take home. Or ask if you can order a half-sized portion at half the cost. Or order with a friend and split the meal. Our family enjoys a Mexican restaurant nearby that serves large entrées along with heaping portions of rice and beans. As soon as my plate arrives, I cut my entrée in half and divide the rice and beans as well. I figure that I can either force myself to eat the entire meal and feel overwhelmingly stuffed, or I can enjoy half the meal and save the rest for lunch the next day.

Another tip our family has discovered is that some restaurants don't have an age limit for children's meals. If you ask, you may be served a smaller portion of food at a lower price. The downside of this is that most of the children's menus are limited in what they offer, and the foods they do offer are usually the high-fat ones such as burgers, hot dogs, and grilled-cheese sandwiches. Even so, if you're trying to gradually change your eating habits, and you aren't ready to give up a burger and fries, ordering the children's meal will at least give you an appropriately sized portion of food.

At fast-food establishments, never "upsize" or order the larger meal. So what if it's a better value for your dollar? It's a terrible value for your body! Think of the healthful foods you need, and reward your body with these instead of punishing it with even more fat.

STRATEGY #2: MASTER MENU MEANINGS

Yes, we all know what the word *fried* means, but what about all those other terms we see on menus? Have you ever thought you were ordering something that was going to be low fat, only to be served a plate heaped with sauce and cheese? It's happened to me many times. Sometimes the menu doesn't specify that the dish is served with cheese, so I wouldn't know to ask for the cheese to be left off. Understanding terms commonly used on menus or in naming dishes will help you anticipate what's going to show up on your plate.

You'll want to avoid foods that use the following words in the name or description:

- *Alfredo:* Cheese-and-cream-based sauce.
- *Au Gratin:* Usually refers to a food covered with cheese or bread-crumbs and butter.
- *Buttery:* This doesn't mean it just tastes like butter; it means there really is butter in it.
- *Creamed, creamy,* or *in cream sauce:* Cream and butter have been added.
- *Crisped:* Any variation of the word crisp generally means fried. The same is true with any variation of the word *fried (pan fried, oven fried, lightly fried).*
- *Hollandaise sauce:* Includes egg yolks and butter. If the name of a sauce ends in *aise,* it's likely to be made with eggs and butter.
- *Sautéed:* Cooked in butter or oil.

If it appears that an unwanted item is added at the end of the cooking process—such as a sauce or a heavy covering of cheese—ask that this item be left off or served on the side. Many unwanted fats and oils are in the sauces and dressings that are poured over foods. These can be easily avoided or used sparingly.

Here are "healthy" terms you want to look for on the menu:

- *Au jus:* This is the drippings or juice from the meat. Usually no fat is added (although it may contain some fat from the meat). This is a better option than gravy.
- *Blanched:* Fresh vegetables can be cooked this way. They're dropped into boiling water, then quickly put into cold water. It's

a quick way of cooking that keeps foods crunchy and can remove unwanted peelings as well. It's a great way to partially cook foods without added fat.

- *Braised:* Braised foods are slowly cooked in a tightly covered pan. Usually, no fat is added. Ask your server to be sure.
- *Grilled:* When meat is grilled over a flame, some of the fat drains away. Vegetables are also tasty when grilled. However, be sure to ask the server if butter is poured over the grilled food or if an oil-based marinade is used. Both of these techniques are common in restaurants and add unwanted fat.
- *Poached:* Generally, poached foods are boiled, steamed, or simmered in water.
- *Roasted:* Usually, roasted foods have been baked, but as with grilled foods, marinades or oils may have been poured over them during the cooking process.

As you can see, even if a food is prepared in a desirable manner, the restaurant can thwart your good intentions by adding butter or oil. I've been disappointed more than once to find my steamed broccoli had been covered with butter before being brought to my table. I've learned that it's very important to ask your server for clarification before ordering. Even if you skip sautéed vegetables and choose grilled ones instead, if the chef ladles a spoonful of oil over the top, your good intentions just went out the window.

STRATEGY #3: PLAN AHEAD

One study showed that people stopped for fast food purely on impulse 70 percent of the time.[10] This means that only 30 percent of the time did consumers say, "Let's take the kids to McDonald's for lunch today." Most of the time they found themselves on the road with a car full of hungry kids—or alone in the car—and pulled into a fast-food joint to grab a bite to eat.

So the first defense against fast-food stops is to figure out how to make them less frequently. When Tony was younger, he would often become thirsty while we were out. It was easy to pull into a drive-through and order him a soft drink. (True, no fat, but it was liquid candy nonetheless.) One day I had the brilliant idea to just bring along a water bottle. That was a no-brainer, right? Even though my water-bottle breakthrough seems obvious in retrospect, we often demonstrate the same lack of planning when we go out the door. We know we're going to be gone for three or four hours, but we don't take along a healthy snack such as fruit or pretzels to tide us over.

Again, there's nothing wrong with eating at a fast-food restaurant, but it's helpful to temper our "impulse buy" with sound information so we don't succumb to the allure of that double cheeseburger, extra-large fries, and triple-thick chocolate shake. When you make unplanned fast-food stops, take a moment at the counter or drive-through menu board to determine what the most healthful food choice will be. Also, keep this question in the forefront of your mind: "Since this meal will be gobbled down in ten minutes, what can I eat that will leave me feeling good about myself an hour from now?"

STRATEGY #4: LEARN THE FACTS ABOUT FAST FOODS

Most restaurants provide nutritional information if you ask for it. You can also find it on their Web sites or by calling their customer service number.

And just so you don't think that restaurants can claim anything simply to persuade you to eat at their establishments, the Food and Drug Administration has published regulations (the Nutrition Labeling and Education Act) stating that claims made about the nutritional values of foods must be true.[11]

Smaller restaurants, or those that aren't part of a national chain, may not have nutritional information available. In these cases, you'll need to communicate with your server and make food choices based on descriptions of items listed on the menu. A little more work, but not impossible.

Let's start by taking a look at fast-food restaurants, scanning the popular menu items to get an idea of which foods are going to give us the most and least fat grams. Since many fast-food restaurants serve pretty much the same menu, even looking at a few of the bigger chains will give you an idea of what to order at similar establishments.

McDonald's

Big Mac: 34 grams of fat

Quarter Pounder: 21 grams of fat

Hamburger: 10 grams of fat

Crispy Chicken: 26 grams of fat

Chicken McGrill with mayonnaise: 18 grams of fat

Chicken McGrill without mayonnaise: 7 grams of fat

Chicken McNuggets (4 pieces): 11 grams of fat

Supersize French Fries: 29 grams of fat

Small French Fries: 10 grams of fat

Garden Salad: 6 grams of fat

Ranch Dressing (one packet): 18 grams of fat

Fat-Free Herb Vinaigrette: 0 grams of fat

Fruit 'n Yogurt Parfait: 5 grams of fat

(Source: www.mcdonalds.com)

As you can see, ordering a grilled chicken sandwich without the mayonnaise is the best way to go. This is true at just about any fast-food restaurant. Some places offer fat-free barbeque sauces, which add flavor to chicken sandwiches. If you don't like your sandwich "dry," try it with ketchup or mustard—both are fat free. Or take your sandwich home, and spread it with your own fat-free mayonnaise.

Were you surprised to see that the chicken nuggets actually have more fat than a regular hamburger? While chicken is generally a good choice, anytime it's fried, it suddenly becomes laden with fat grams.

What would make a nutritious and filling meal at McDonald's? Try a grilled chicken sandwich without the mayo, or a garden salad with fat-free dressing, and add a Fruit 'n Yogurt Parfait for dessert.

Wendy's

Big Bacon Classic: 29 grams of fat

Classic Single with Everything: 19 grams of fat

Jr. Hamburger: 9 grams of fat

Chicken Club Sandwich: 19 grams of fat

Grilled Chicken Sandwich: 7 grams of fat

Great Biggie French Fries: 23 grams of fat

Medium French Fries: 17 grams of fat

Plain Baked Potato: 0 grams of fat

Hot Stuffed Baked Potato with Sour Cream and Chives: 6 grams of fat

Caesar Side Salad (plain): 4 grams of fat

Mandarin Chicken Salad (plain): 1.5 grams of fat

Small Chili: 6 grams of fat

Small Frosty: 8 grams of fat

(Source: www.wendys.com)

Again, choosing foods other than the burgers will give you a filling meal without as much fat. A plain baked potato doesn't have a lot of flavor, and since the portion of sour cream is small, an excessive amount of fat is not added with the sour cream and chives option. If you're really hungry, top your baked potato with a small chili—lots of flavor and plenty of food without too much fat.

Wendy's also serves an array of salads. Unfortunately, most of them have cheese and other high-fat toppings, such as sour cream, chips, fried noodles, nuts, and so on. Choose a salad with the fewest of these toppings and more vegetables. Ask for a fat-free dressing.

Subway

Meatball Sandwich: 26 grams of fat

Tuna Sandwich: 22 grams of fat

Sweet Onion Chicken Teriyaki: 5 grams of fat

Turkey Breast: 4.5 grams of fat

Turkey Breast and Ham: 5 grams of fat

Veggie Delite: 3 grams of fat

Oatmeal Raisin Cookie: 8 grams of fat

*All information is for six-inch sandwiches.

(Source: www.subway.com)

In their advertisements, Subway has made a big deal about people who have lost large amounts of weight by eating at their restaurants. They're one of the few fast-food chains that offer a variety of vegetables for their sandwiches and don't add extra fat without your permission. Leaving off the optional cheese, mayonnaise, special dressings, and oil still leaves a sandwich piled high with nutritious and delicious fillings. Ask for all the veggies you can get, and you won't go away hungry.

Notice that the tuna sandwich is fairly high in fat, especially when compared to other options at Subway. Most people think they're making a good choice when they opt for fish, but they forget to consider how the fish is prepared. As with chicken, frying will always add a lot of fat to this normally low-fat food, as will adding mayonnaise. When you make tuna sandwiches at home, you can always use fat-free mayonnaise. And sometimes smaller, family-owned or local restaurants have the ability to make tuna or chicken salad to order with fat-free products.

Schlotzsky's Deli

The Original (regular): 31 grams of fat

Large Original (family size): 58 grams of fat

Chicken Breast Sandwich (regular): 4 grams of fat

Pesto Chicken Sandwich (regular): 9 grams of fat

Turkey Original (regular): 32 grams of fat

Smoked Turkey Breast (regular): 7 grams of fat

Albacore Tuna Sandwich (regular): 10 grams of fat

Vegetarian Sandwich (regular): 11 grams of fat

Thai Chicken Pizza (8-inch): 17 grams of fat

California Pasta Salad: 3 grams of fat

Garden Salad (plain): 1 gram of fat

Sesame Ginger Vinaigrette: 15 grams of fat

(Source: www.schlotzskys.com)

When I realized how low in fat many of the sandwiches were at Subway, I mistakenly thought the same would be true of any deli that made fresh sandwiches. The first time I researched the nutritional information for Schlotzsky's, I thought there was a misprint. A number of their sandwiches had over 70 grams of fat, with a couple even having 97 and 98 grams of fat. I realized that by adding oil-based sauces, cheese, olives, and plenty of meat, many of the sandwiches I'd been ordering were not good choices. Fortunately, Schlotzsky's has since lowered the fat in their sandwiches, and they do offer several flavorful low-fat alternatives—just be sure to skip the oil-based sauces and the cheese.

Taco Bell

Taco: 12 grams of fat

Taco Supreme: 16 grams of fat

Chicken Soft Taco: 7 grams of fat

Bean Burrito: 12 grams of fat

7-Layer Burrito: 22 grams of fat

Nachos: 18 grams of fat

Pintos 'n Cheese: 8 grams of fat

Mexican Rice: 9 grams of fat

(Source: www.tacobell.com)

It's tricky to get a filling and low-fat meal at Taco Bell and other similar fast-food restaurants because most of the tortillas are fried, cheese is used to top almost every menu item, and sour cream and guacamole are added to many foods as well. The chicken soft taco is a good choice, but eating one taco doesn't satisfy most people. Choose foods using flour tortillas that are not fried rather than the corn tortillas that are always fried. Since Taco Bell prepares the food after you order it, stick with items that use beans and chicken, and request that the cheese and sour cream be left off.

Pizza Hut

Cheese with Hand-Tossed Crust: 10 grams of fat

Cheese with a Pan Pizza Crust: 14 grams of fat

Cheese with Thin 'n Crispy Crust: 9 grams of fat

Pepperoni with Hand-Tossed Crust: 13 grams of fat

Veggie Lover's with Hand-Tossed Crust: 8 grams of fat

Chicken Supreme with Hand-Tossed Crust: 7 grams of fat

Spaghetti with Marinara Sauce: 6 grams of fat

*Information is for one slice of a medium-size pizza.

(Source: www.pizzahut.com)

Pizza gets a bad rap. If you load it with veggies and go easy on the cheese, it's not a bad fast-food option. The problem is, most people have trouble stopping at one piece of pizza. For a filling meal, try a slice of the Veggie Lover's or Chicken Supreme pizza, accompanied by a salad with fat-free dressing or an order of spaghetti. Lower the fat by asking for your pizza to have extra vegetables (except for olives) and less cheese, and you can have an extra slice.

Note the difference in fat that occurs when you change the thickness of the crust. The thinnest crust does trim off a gram or two with each slice, but it also may not leave you feeling satisfied. The thickest crust is, unfortunately, cooked in a pan coated with butter (almost fried) to get that crispy bottom, so it has more fat. With the hand-tossed crust, you'll get a serving of grains and not a lot of extra fat.

KFC

Original Recipe Chicken Breast: 24 grams of fat

Extra Crispy Chicken Breast: 28 grams of fat

Tender Roast Sandwich without sauce: 5 grams of fat

Honey BBQ-Flavored Sandwich: 6 grams of fat

Colonel's Crispy Strips (3 strips): 16 grams of fat

Mashed Potatoes with Gravy: 6 grams of fat

Corn on the Cob: 1.5 grams of fat

BBQ Baked Beans: 3 grams of fat

Green Beans: 1.5 grams of fat

Mean Greens: 3 grams of fat

Little Bucket Parfait—Strawberry Shortcake: 7 grams of fat

(Source: www.kfc.com)

It was no mistake when Kentucky Fried Chicken changed their name to KFC. They knew people wanted lower-fat foods and having the word *fried* right in the middle of their name didn't help matters. Fortunately, they didn't just change their name; they also made adjustments to their menu so that it's easy to find a low-fat meal that's tasty and filling.

KFC offers several sandwiches and vegetable side dishes that are low in fat. You could make a whole meal of side dishes, get all those wonderful nutrients from vegetables, and still be filled with low-fat foods. But be sure to skip the mayonnaise-based coleslaw and potato salad. Even though they have plenty of veggies in them, they also have lots of fat.

The Grocery Store

Amazingly, few of us consider the grocery store when we're hungry and need a quick bite. Markets are usually just as easy to find as fast-food places (although I've never seen one with a drive-through window). Take the trouble to get out of your car and walk inside to grab a roll from the bakery and several pieces of fruit or vegetables. Wash your meal down with bottled water or a carton of cold juice, and you've just had the ultimate fast food.

STRATEGY #5: BE SAVVY IN CHINESE, MEXICAN, AND ITALIAN RESTAURANTS

It is usually a pleasure to dine out at "real" restaurants (ones that serve beverages in glasses rather than paper cups and don't wrap your food in paper). Whether you're celebrating a special event, meeting a dear friend, or just want to get away from the kitchen for a while, sitting down to a fully prepared meal is a treat.

Before you follow the host or hostess to your table, however, be sure you've thought about what foods will give you maximum nutrition and minimum fat. Some chains offer nutritional information at their establishments or through their main offices. Others have made low-fat dining easier by placing an icon such as a heart or a piece of fruit beside menu items that are lower in fat or calories. These icons might actually signify a low-fat food, or they might denote foods that are simply lower in fat than the general fare. Be careful! When you don't have access to the facts, use wise judgment and the information from this chapter to help you make the best choices.

People are often confused when dining at restaurants that serve foods from other countries, as menu items and ingredients aren't always familiar. Cooking methods may differ from ones we're accustomed to, and your server may not even speak your language fluently. If possible, research the ethnic foods you enjoy to learn which ones are prepared with oils and fatty meats and which are not. Since Chinese, Mexican, and Italian restaurants are popular, let's look at what foods are generally the best to eat and the ones that are the best to avoid at these restaurants.

Chinese Restaurants

One study found that more than half of Americans considered Chinese food "more healthful" than other foods they normally ate.[12] But many foods at Chinese restaurants are fried, cooked with pork, have nuts added, and sometimes are deep-fried first, then stir-fried.

Begin by choosing steamed rice instead of fried rice, and allow yourself plenty of it. Fried rice is cooked in oil, and usually has eggs in it. Some establishments add pork as well. Steamed rice has less than .5 grams of fat per serving. And when you eat a larger portion of rice with a smaller portion of a meat-based dish as a topping, you'll eat less fat.

Along with rice, look for dishes with lots of vegetables. As with rice, choose steamed vegetables instead of stir-fried. If steamed vegetables aren't available, stir-fried may be the best option you have at a Chinese restaurant. Any dish that has a high proportion of vegetables will be better than a meat-based dish. For example, select vegetable lo mein over the kind made with chicken, beef, or pork. Ask for broth-based soups and ones that have tofu as the base.

Avoid menu items that are fried or made with nuts. Kung Pao chicken, Mu Shu pork, sweet and sour pork or chicken, and egg rolls are all fried, as are many other dishes. Any food with a crispy coating is deep-fried or stir-fried and will be loaded with extra fat. As for the nuts, Kung Pao chicken, cashew chicken, and sesame chicken are best avoided.

Mexican Restaurants

As we saw with our survey of the Taco Bell menu, many foods in Mexican restaurants use fried tortillas and are topped with cheese, sour cream, and guacamole. Don't be discouraged, however, as there are plenty of tasty, healthy options at Mexican restaurants.

Select menu items that use flour tortillas that are not fried, such as burritos, and find items that feature grilled vegetables, black beans, and rice. Ask how the rice and beans are cooked. These may have been prepared in lard, but many restaurants are now offering a lower-fat option of beans and rice cooked with broth or other flavorings instead of oil.

Fajitas are usually prepared fresh, right when you order. Request that your dish (usually made with plenty of veggies) be prepared with less oil. Then mix the vegetables with a reasonable portion of rice.

A popular item at Mexican restaurants is a salad served inside a fried tortilla bowl. Eat the salad and leave the bowl behind. Or ask for the same salad to be served in a regular bowl.

Request that cheese, sour cream, and guacamole be left off, or ask if the restaurant offers a low-fat alternative. Some restaurants do have fat-free sour cream if you ask, and one chain has a lower-fat cheese available as well.

Salsas are almost always fat free, made with fresh vegetables and spices. You can pour as much as you like over your flour tortilla, rice, and beans.

Italian Restaurants

My friend Tricia grew up in Italy and says the food there looks almost nothing like the Americanized versions served here. They eat a lot more fresh fruits and vegetables with their pasta and bread, and less of the meats and cheeses that we add in abundance. Let's follow the Italians' lead.

Pasta, like rice, is one of those grains you can eat plenty of. If your pasta is not drenched in oil or butter, you can eat till you're full. However, most of us don't like plain pasta, and this is where there's more good news. There are many Italian sauces that are low in fat. Tomato sauce, marinara sauce, and red clam sauce are good lower-fat options. Skip the meat, cheese, and cream-based sauces, and stick to those that are heavy on the tomatoes.

Soups and salads are often served in Italian restaurants, so be sure to choose broth-based soups (such as minestrone) or veggie-full soups. Vegetable salads can be a great option if you ask for fat-free dressing or at least have the dressing served on the side so you can use just a small amount.

Bread is a mainstay at Italian restaurants, and this *can* be a low-fat food. Ask for breadsticks that have not been coated with butter, then dip them in your tomato-based sauce instead. The same goes for your vegetables. Request that they be served either steamed or grilled and without cheese or butter.

As with every other restaurant, pass over the foods that are fried. Eggplant parmesan is breaded and fried and covered with cheese. Veal or chicken piccata is cooked in oil as well. Read the menu carefully to see which foods are prepared with oil.

The worst dishes in terms of fat content are the ones with cream and cheese, such as lasagna, fettuccine Alfredo, and cheese manicotti. Lasagna can be made with vegetables instead of meat, but restaurants are still generous with cheeses.

STRATEGY #6: BE PREPARED FOR DINNER
AT A FRIEND'S HOUSE

"Can you join us for dinner?"

While pursuing the Low-Fat Lifestyle, no one wants to decline the gracious invitation of friends for dinner at their house. We joke that Mike is a "high-maintenance friend" because he can have almost no fat in his diet, so it's often hard for people to figure out what to offer him. Even though it's sometimes awkward to ask friends what will be served, it's necessary for his health. But he almost gets off easy here because it is necessary for him to ask. What about the rest of us who want to eat healthy but wouldn't actually get sick if a cheesy dish were served?

Once when we were eating with friends at their home, our hostess gladly set aside vegetables and rice for Mike, then poured butter and cheese on top of what the rest of us would eat. Because I hadn't made my preferences known, she assumed I didn't mind having the extra fat.

So how *do* we tactfully request that our host or hostess not serve fatty foods?

To be honest, it's sometimes awkward and difficult. You don't want to risk offending the host or creating hassles for the cook. Yet it's your body, and you have the right to make healthy food choices. If you were at a friend's home and she offered you a cigarette, you would have no trouble declining. You'd simply say, "No, thanks." But when that friend hands you a slice of chocolate pie, you feel obligated to eat every last crumb.

Take heart, we have a few options. First, be honest with the host or hostess from the beginning. When you're invited to dine at someone's home, give a clear and simple statement of your eating habits. Say, "Thank you for the invitation! I'd love to join you on that date but want to let you know about my diet restrictions. I am avoiding most meats and other high-fat foods. If this will be too much hassle for you, I'd be glad to bring a dish to add to the table." This allows your friend the choice of either preparing foods that you can eat or letting you bring something along.

I'll warn you, though, this plan is not fail-safe. I recently became acquainted with some of Mike's friends from high school, and we invited them to join us for lunch. The wife graciously offered to bring a home-made pecan pie for dessert. I knew this would be filled with fat, so without any explanation, I suggested that a fruit salad would probably be a better idea. She gladly agreed. Well, when they walked into our house, she handed me a lovely glass bowl filled with her fruit salad—made of whipped cream, cream cheese, a whole bag of miniature marshmallows, maraschino cherries, and a few grapes and pineapple chunks. It was a beautiful salad, but not the array of fresh fruits I'd had in mind!

We served the salad, and everyone enjoyed it. As this woman and I got better acquainted, we could joke about the "nutritious" salad-dessert she'd brought. Fortunately, I had plenty of low-fat foods to serve as well. The point is, you may find yourself in a similar predicament if you're not honest and direct with your friends.

A second option is to simply go along and hope you're served nutritious foods or eat small portions if only butter-drenched and cheese-coated foods are served. I've done this when I couldn't avoid it and just had very small servings. I didn't starve, and I remembered to bring along a few low-fat items the next time.

A third option you can try is to politely decline foods that aren't going to satisfy your healthful desires. There's no sin in saying, "That looks delicious, but I'd better pass. Thanks anyway." No further explanation is required. Eat the vegetables and the pasta or rice, and pass the meat on to the next person. Then when dessert is served, politely decline or ask if you might have a piece of fruit instead. If these people are truly your friends, they won't be offended. If they are offended, they'll get over it. It's not your responsibility to eat foods out of guilt or the fear of hurting someone else's feelings.

One last option we rarely consider is to redirect the invitation so that it doesn't involve a meal. Eating together is a social activity, but there are other ways to spend time together that don't revolve around food. Ask your friend to join you for a walk instead of brunch. You can talk as you tour an art gallery or browse through a craft store just as you can while you eat a sandwich. Put your creative mind to use and think of other things you can do with friends that don't mean you'll need to eat together.

No matter where you're dining—at home, in a restaurant, or in someone else's home—you're sure to find many foods that will be nutritious, delicious, and hassle free. Keep on with this adventure, and you'll find it's not as tricky as you thought.

FIVE

Recipes for Low-Fat Eating

From the fullness of his grace we have all received one blessing after another.

—JOHN 1:16

My family jokes about my mother's cooking. Mom is a wonderful
cook, always trying new dishes or looking for ways to improve upon the
standards. Most of the time we love to eat whatever she makes. But she
sometimes takes experimenting a little too far. One time she made a
pumpkin pie—using puréed pinto beans instead of pumpkin! She assured
us that it tasted just like pumpkin pie. She was right that it had enough
cinnamon and cloves, but there was no way to mask the thick pastiness of
the pinto beans. Yuck!

You'll be relieved to know *that* recipe is not included in these pages.
(Sorry, Mom!) Instead, you'll find recipes that are easy to prepare, are kid-
and family-tested, and are accompanied by helpful tips and comments.

Many of the dishes combine foods from several of the food groups.
For example, the recipe for Chicken and Rice Soup contains poultry, a
grain, and vegetables. So the recipes aren't easily divided into sections like
meat, vegetables, and grain. Instead, I've organized them according to category: main dishes, additional vegetable or fruit dishes, and so on.

With each recipe, I've included an estimate of the amount of fat in each serving. This will vary slightly as you cook, since you may choose, say, a brand of pasta with more or less fat than the brand I chose. And as chicken breasts are not all the same size, it's impossible to know the exact amount of fat your recipe will have without weighing every single item. The figures I've included are based on standard products and average sizes of readily available foods. Be sure to read the labels on the foods you purchase, and prepare to get a more accurate accounting of the grams of fat per serving.

Grab your favorite apron, and let's get cooking!

MAIN DISHES

Chicken and Rice Soup

This soup makes a delicious main dish. And when you're in need of home-made chicken soup to fight the sniffles, this is an excellent choice.

2 boneless, skinless chicken breasts
2 cups fat-free chicken broth
1 cup chopped carrot
1 cup chopped onion
1 cup chopped celery
¼ teaspoon oregano
¼ teaspoon black pepper
½ cup uncooked rice

Cut chicken into bite-size chunks, and simmer in chicken broth. Add in vegetables and spices and water as needed to cover the vegetables and meat. Cook over low heat until the vegetables are tender and the chicken is cooked through. Add rice and cook 30 minutes more, adding water as needed.

Serves: 4

Approximate grams of fat per serving: 3

Black Bean Soup

Serve this with baked tortilla chips. A splash of lime juice gives added zip to this soup. To make a side dish of black beans, reduce the water to 1 cup and after simmering, just mash the beans a little with a potato masher. It's a great meal when you make Mexican rice and these beans together. Very tasty!

½ medium-size onion, finely chopped
¼ cup white cooking wine or water
¼ teaspoon dried garlic
2 teaspoons chili powder
1 teaspoon ground cumin
2 cans black beans, rinsed and drained
2 chicken bouillon cubes
1 cup water

Simmer onion in the wine or water for about 5 minutes or until tender. Stir in garlic, chili powder, and cumin. Cook only 30 seconds. Add in beans, bouillon cubes, and 2 cups of water. Heat to boiling, then turn down heat and simmer, uncovered, for 15 minutes.

Pour the entire mixture into your blender. Leave lid on loosely to let steam escape, and turn blender off and on quickly one or two times. Don't purée or leave the blender on. Pour back into the pan and keep warm until you're ready to serve.

Serves: 4

Approximate grams of fat per serving: 3.5

Chicken Stew

You can add any variety of vegetables to this stew. It's an ideal way to use leftover veggies of any kind. I've added chopped spinach, celery, and even leftover mashed potatoes.

2 boneless, skinless chicken breasts

1 large potato

1 box (10 ounces) frozen mixed vegetables

½ cup chopped onion

1 can (15 ounces) tomato sauce

1 teaspoon Worcestershire sauce

Salt and pepper to taste

Cut chicken into bite-size chunks. Peel and chop the potato. Place chicken, potato, vegetables, and onion in a large pot. Add just enough water to cover them. Simmer over medium heat until the potato is tender. Add tomato sauce and Worcestershire sauce, and season with salt and pepper.

Serves: 4

Approximate grams of fat per serving: 3.5

Baked Potato Soup

This tastes like a baked potato, but with the filling warmth of soup. Great on a cold winter evening!

3 large potatoes

1 onion, chopped

1 can skim evaporated milk

½ teaspoon black pepper

4 strips extra lean turkey bacon

½ cup fat-free cheddar cheese

½ cup fat-free sour cream

Cut potatoes into bite-size chunks—you can peel the potatoes or leave the skin on as you like. Put potato and onion into a pan, and add just enough water to cover the potatoes. Boil gently until potatoes are done.

Drain off a little of the water, then add canned milk and pepper. Use a potato masher to mash the potato slightly so that the soup is thick and chunky. Keep warm until ready to serve, but don't bring it to a boil.

Ladle soup into bowls and top each with sour cream, cheese, and a strip of crumbled bacon.

Serves: 4

Approximate grams of fat per serving: less than 1

Variation: You can add any vegetables you like to this soup before adding milk. Broccoli, cauliflower, celery, and carrots add good flavor and texture. Or try something new!

Green Chili

2 cans (2 ounces) pinto beans, rinsed and drained

2 boneless, skinless chicken breasts

1 can (4 ounces) mild chopped green chilies

1 teaspoon ground cumin

½ teaspoon oregano

¼ teaspoon ground cloves

½ teaspoon garlic powder

½ cup chopped onion

2 cans fat-free chicken broth

Cut chicken into bite-size chunks. Mix all ingredients in a large pot and bring to a boil. Then simmer over low heat for about 30 minutes.

Serves: 4

Approximate grams of fat per serving: 3.5

Variation: White, skinless turkey can also be used in any recipe calling for chicken.

Chicken and Broccoli Casserole

Many people who aren't big fans of broccoli are won over by this creamy dish. For extra flavor, cook the rice in fat-free chicken broth or add a chicken bouillon cube to the water as the rice cooks.

2 boneless, skinless chicken breasts

1 ½ pounds fresh or frozen broccoli

1 can (10 ounces) low-fat cream of chicken soup (or low-fat cream of
*   mushroom, depending on your tastes)*

¼ cup fat-free mayonnaise

2 tablespoons lemon juice

½ cup skim milk

½ teaspoon garlic powder

⅛ teaspoon Italian seasoning

1 cup fat-free cheddar cheese

2 cups cooked rice

Prepare your casserole dish by lightly coating it with nonstick cooking spray. Spread cooked rice in the bottom of this dish. Cut chicken into bite-size chunks. Lightly coat skillet with nonstick cooking spray, then brown chicken in the skillet.

Cook broccoli in microwave or steam on stovetop until tender. Drain broccoli and spoon over rice. Spoon chicken over broccoli and rice mixture.

Mix the soup, mayonnaise, lemon juice, milk, garlic powder, and Italian seasoning in a separate bowl, and spread over other ingredients in casserole. Top with grated cheese. Bake at 350 degrees for about 30 minutes.

Serves: 6

Approximate grams of fat per serving: 3

"Fried" Chicken

This dish offers the taste of fried chicken nuggets without very much added fat.

3 boneless, skinless, chicken breasts

½ cup flour

½ teaspoon black pepper

1 tablespoon butter

Cut chicken into nugget-size chunks. Mix flour and pepper, then dredge chicken in the flour mixture so each piece is coated. Melt butter in a frying pan, and add chicken pieces. Cook for several minutes on medium to high heat, then turn chicken over, being careful not to let chicken burn. Serve with rice or pasta.

Serves: 4

Approximate grams of fat per serving: 7.5

Shredded Chicken BBQ

This dish is easy to make ahead of time—and quite tasty as a light summer meal.

2 boneless, skinless chicken breasts
1 cup fat-free BBQ sauce, store-bought
4 low-fat hamburger buns

Place chicken in an oven-safe covered dish. Pour sauce over chicken; cover dish and place in oven. Cook at 350 degrees for 30 to 45 minutes or until the meat is done. Use two forks to shred the meat. Add more BBQ sauce to taste. Serve on buns.

Serves: 4

Approximate grams of fat per serving: 5

Cooking Tip: Save time with chicken dishes by cooking the chicken in a crock pot during the day. When you're ready to prepare your meal, the chicken will be ready to chop or shred.

Shredded Chicken Tacos

2 boneless, skinless chicken breasts
½ cup water
1 packet powdered taco seasoning

8 taco shells
Chopped tomato
Chopped lettuce
Fat-free sour cream
Fat-free cheddar cheese
Fat-free salsa

Place chicken in an oven-safe covered dish. Add ½ cup water. Cover dish and place in oven. Cook at 350 degrees for 30 to 45 minutes or until the meat is done. Use two forks to shred chicken. Add the taco seasoning and more water as needed. Serve chicken in taco shells with tomatoes, lettuce, sour cream, cheese, and salsa to taste.

Serves: 4

Approximate grams of fat per serving: 7

Time Tip: The chicken can also be prepared in a crock pot.

Mexican Chicken Casserole

This recipe is a great way to use leftover tortilla chips. Even stale chips can be used and will taste fine. For a different flavor, leave out the green chilies and the milk, and add a can of RO-TEL or chopped tomatoes with Mexican seasonings instead.

2 boneless, skinless chicken breasts
1 can (10 ounces) low-fat cream of chicken soup
½ cup fat-free sour cream
1 can (4 ounces) diced green chilies

½ cup chopped green onions
½ teaspoon garlic powder
½ cup skim milk
6 ounces baked tortilla chips (about half a bag)
1 cup fat-free cheddar cheese

Cut chicken into bite-size chunks. Brown chicken in skillet lightly coated with nonstick cooking spray. Place meat in a bowl and add soup, skim milk, sour cream, green chilies, green onions, and garlic. Stir until mixed. Spread tortilla chips in bottom of a casserole dish and gently crush. Pour chicken mixture on top of chips, and cover with cheese. Bake at 350 degrees for 20 to 30 minutes.

Serves: 6

Approximate grams of fat per serving: 4

Cajun Chicken and Pasta

You can adjust the spiciness of this dish to your own tastes by adding more Cajun seasoning. If you serve this as a leftover, add a little skim milk since the pasta will have absorbed the sauce during storage.

2 boneless, skinless chicken breasts
1 green or red pepper, cut into narrow strips (or you can use half of each
    for a different flavor and more color)
4 large mushrooms, sliced (optional)
½ cup chopped onion
½ cup water or white cooking wine
1 can skim evaporated milk

2 teaspoons Cajun seasoning

¼ teaspoon dried basil

¼ teaspoon garlic powder

¼ teaspoon pepper

6 ounces linguine, cooked and drained

Cut chicken into bite-size chunks. Brown chicken in skillet lightly coated with nonstick cooking spray. Add peppers, mushrooms, and onion. Add ½ cup water or white cooking wine. Cook on medium heat until vegetables are tender and liquid is absorbed, then add milk and all the other seasonings. Cook over low heat for a few minutes to let seasonings blend. (Don't boil once milk has been added.) Mix in the linguine and serve.

Serves: 4

Approximate grams of fat per serving: 4

Meat Pies

The mixture of meat and spices usually associated with baking is an unusual and tasty treat. The generic brand of onion soup mix is less expensive than the name brands and tastes just as good.

½ Yeast Roll recipe (see Bread section)

1 pound extra lean ground turkey (99 percent fat free)

1 package onion soup mix

1 teaspoon cinnamon

½ teaspoon nutmeg

½ teaspoon cloves

½ teaspoon garlic powder

½ cup water

Make yeast dough and set aside. Brown ground turkey and stir in soup mix and all spices. Add about ½ cup of water and stir until everything is mixed and coated with seasonings. Cook on medium heat for a couple of minutes so that some of the water cooks off, and the entire mixture looks tender but not dry.

Take a handful of dough—about the amount you'd use to make one roll—and form a ball. Place on a floured surface, and use a rolling pin to roll dough into a circle bigger than your outstretched fingers. Put a heaping spoonful of meat filling into the center of the dough. Pinch the edges of the dough together securely so no filling shows. Repeat until all of the dough and filling have been used.

Place pastries on a cooking sheet that's been lightly coated with non-stick cooking spray, and bake at 350 degrees for about 15 to 20 minutes or until dough is lightly browned. Serve hot.

Serves: 8

Approximate grams of fat per serving: 1.5

Variations: Taco Meat Pie—For a little extra spice, try substituting a package of taco seasoning for the onion soup mix and spices. After the meat pie is cooked, split open a side and stuff with fat-free grated cheese, chopped tomatoes, and any other taco toppings you like, such as fat-free sour cream or salsa.

Pizza Meat Pie—Instead of filling dough with a turkey-and-spice mixture, place a spoonful of low-fat store-bought spaghetti sauce on the dough, and add grated fat-free mozzarella cheese and whatever pizza toppings you like (such as turkey pepperoni, onions, or peppers). It is very important that the dough for these pies be sealed completely, as the sauce will seep out during cooking.

RICE AND PASTA

"Fried" Rice

Serve with steamed vegetables or baked chicken with a soy-sauce marinade.

> ½ cup chopped green pepper
> ½ cup chopped red pepper
> ¼ cup chopped mushroom
> Egg substitute to equal 1 egg
> 2 cups cooked rice
> 2 tablespoons soy sauce

Coat skillet with nonstick cooking spray, and sauté the vegetables until just tender. Add the egg substitute, and stir constantly until egg is cooked, cutting egg into tiny pieces. Add rice and soy sauce, and stir over low heat until thoroughly heated.

Serves: 4

Approximate grams of fat per serving: less than .5

Mexican Rice

This is an easy side dish—great with Mexican food, or serve it with Black Bean Soup for a complete meal.

> ⅓ cup chopped onion (or more if you like a lot of onion)
> ⅓ cup chopped green pepper
> 1 cup uncooked rice (not instant)
> 2 tablespoons white wine

1 can (15 ounces) chopped tomatoes (if you like a little more flavor, get
*   the kind with chilies in them)*
Dash of black pepper
1 teaspoon Worcestershire sauce
½ teaspoon mustard (the kind you put on sandwiches—not the dried spice)
1 beef bouillon cube
1 cup water

Sauté onion and green pepper in white wine until tender. Add rice and stir over medium heat for 1 minute. Add remaining ingredients along with 1 cup of water. Bring to a boil, then reduce heat and cover. Cook 20 to 30 minutes, until rice is tender and the liquid is absorbed. Stir a few times in the cooking process to make sure rice doesn't burn.

Serves: 4

Approximate grams of fat per serving: less than .5

Fettuccine with Capers

This dish surprised me because the pasta was so tender and tasty, yet it didn't have a heavy sauce. Capers are pea-shaped flower buds from a Mediterranean bush that are similar in taste to olives. If you don't care for capers, the pasta is still flavorful without them.

1 pound fettuccine
1 can fat-free chicken broth
½ cup white cooking wine
2 tablespoons lemon juice
2 tablespoons drained capers

Cook pasta in water according to directions on package. When it is tender, drain and return pasta to cooking pan. In a smaller pan mix broth, wine, and lemon juice. Bring to a boil, then pour over pasta. Add capers and let simmer for 10 minutes or until ready to serve.

Serves: 4

Approximate grams of fat per serving: 2

Pasta Salad

Experiment with other vegetables in this salad, such as chopped broccoli or zucchini, or add halved cherry tomatoes.

2 cups macaroni

2 carrots, grated

1 cup halved snow peas

¼ cup chopped green onion

½ cup chopped red pepper

Dressing:

½ cup fat-free mayonnaise

½ cup fat-free sour cream

1 tablespoon red wine vinegar

½ teaspoon ground ginger

Pepper to taste

Prepare macaroni according to directions on package. Drain macaroni and mix with vegetables. Whisk together dressing ingredients, and pour over pasta and vegetables. Stir until the salad is coated with dressing. Cover and refrigerate at least 2 hours.

Serves: 4

Approximate grams of fat per serving: less than 1

MORE VEGETABLES

Italian Zucchini

½ cup fat-free chicken broth or white cooking wine

½ cup chopped onion

2 cloves chopped garlic

4 medium zucchini, cut into chunks

¼ teaspoon basil

½ teaspoon oregano

1 can (15 ounces) diced tomatoes

1 can (15 ounces) tomato sauce

Cook onion and garlic in broth or wine on medium heat until onion is tender. Add zucchini, basil, and oregano and cook on medium about 10 minutes, stirring often. Add tomatoes, along with juice from the can, and tomato sauce. Simmer and stir until zucchini is the desired tenderness.

Serves: 6

Approximate grams of fat per serving: 0

Chilled Asparagus

My grandmother, who loves cold asparagus, showed me this easy recipe. You can also use canned asparagus for an even faster dish.

1 pound asparagus spears

½ cup fat-free Italian dressing

Steam asparagus spears until tender. Cool. Place asparagus in a shallow dish and coat with dressing. Refrigerate 2 hours, mixing dressing over the asparagus every 30 minutes. Drain off the dressing, and serve asparagus cold.

Serves: 4

Approximate grams of fat per serving: less than .5

Creamy Cucumbers

If you want a little more color and crunch in your salad, leave the peel on the cucumbers.

> *2 cucumbers, thinly sliced*
> *1 small onion, thinly sliced*
> *½ cup fat-free sour cream*
> *1 tablespoon vinegar*
> *1 teaspoon sugar*

Stir together all ingredients. Cover and chill until ready to serve.

Serves: 4

Approximate grams of fat per serving: 0

Hash Browns

The first time I tried to make hash browns, I didn't know that I should boil the potatoes first. My hash browns turned out gooey and a grayish-purple color. My family was polite and covered them with tons of ketchup before trying to choke them down. Here's the right way to make them:

3 large potatoes
Salt and pepper to taste

Peel the potatoes and cut them in half. Boil potatoes in water for about 10 to 15 minutes. Potatoes should be only partially cooked. Drain and let cool a little. Grate the potatoes and immediately drop them into a pan that's been coated with nonstick cooking spray. Add salt and pepper to taste. Cook on medium heat about 5 minutes, then turn potatoes over with a spatula—they'll fall apart, but turning works better than stirring. Turn every 5 minutes or so until they look brown and crispy.

If you like onion in your hash browns, cook a few tablespoons of chopped onion in chicken broth or white wine before adding the grated potatoes.

Serves: 4

Approximate grams of fat per serving: 0

Cooking Tip: If you don't want to take the time to grate the potatoes, cut them into chunks and follow the recipe—they'll come out shaped a little differently but will still taste great.

French Fries

The egg white in this recipe helps the potatoes brown and crisp without adding fat. Get out the ketchup!

3 large potatoes
2 egg whites
¼ teaspoon garlic powder

½ teaspoon salt

1 tablespoon Parmesan cheese

Peel potatoes and cut into fry-size strips. In a large bowl mix egg whites, garlic, salt, and cheese. Beat lightly with a fork or wire whisk until slightly foamy. Add potatoes and stir or toss until potatoes are thoroughly coated with the egg mixture. Coat a baking pan with nonstick cooking spray. Place potatoes on pan, spreading them evenly over the pan. Bake at 375 degrees for 40 minutes, turning potatoes every 10 minutes.

Serves: 4

Approximate grams of fat per serving: less than .5

BREADS

Yeast Rolls

Who can resist the aroma of fresh bread? Not anyone in my family—and probably not yours, either. They'll love this recipe.

1 package dry yeast

¼ cup very warm water (110 to 115 degrees)

2 cups skim milk

2 tablespoons sugar or honey

1 tablespoon vegetable shortening

2 teaspoons salt

5 to 6 cups of flour

Pour yeast into warm water, and let it sit for about 5 minutes to soften. Warm the milk, sugar, shortening, and salt over low heat, stirring constantly until the shortening is slightly melted (115 to 120 degrees). (You can also do this step in the microwave, checking the temperature of the milk often.)

Pour milk mixture into a large bowl, and add 2 cups of the flour. Beat until mixed, then add the softened yeast. Beat for 2 minutes on high speed. Stir in as much of the remaining flour as you can, then turn the mixture onto a lightly floured surface and knead for about 5 minutes, or until the dough is smooth and elastic. Place the ball of dough into a clean bowl that has been lightly coated with nonstick cooking spray. Cover with a clean cloth, and place in a warm spot. Let the dough rise for 1 hour.

Punch down the dough, cover it again, and let it rest for 10 minutes. Shape the dough into small balls, and place on a baking sheet that's lightly coated with nonstick cooking spray. Cover and let rise again for 45 minutes. Bake at 375 degrees for 10 to 15 minutes, or until rolls are lightly browned.

Serves: 18

Approximate grams of fat per serving: 1

Variations: Bread—This recipe can also be used to make two loaves of bread. After letting the dough rest for 10 minutes, divide and place into two loaf pans that have been lightly coated with nonstick cooking spray. Let rise 45 minutes to 1 hour, then bake at 375 degrees for 45 minutes. Turn loaves from pan and let cool on a wire rack.

Cinnamon Rolls—Roll dough into a rectangle that's about ¼ inch thick. Spread ½ to ¾ cup fat-free sour cream over dough. Mix 2 tablespoons of ground cinnamon with 1 cup of light brown sugar, and sprinkle this over the sour cream. Roll dough out, and cut into slices that are about 2 inches wide. Place rolls into a 9- × 3-inch pan that's been lightly coated with nonstick cooking spray. Cover with a cloth, and let rise for about 1 hour. Bake at 375 degrees for 10 to 15 minutes, or until the rolls are lightly browned and no longer doughy in the center. I don't know whether these are good cold—they never last that long at our house!

Pumpkin Bread

This bread makes a nice gift during the holidays. Or serve it at a brunch, and you won't feel guilty about having two slices! This recipe makes two medium-size loaves or three small ones.

2 cups sugar

1 cup oil replacement or equivalent

6 egg whites or egg substitute to equal 3 eggs

2 cups pumpkin, canned or fresh

3 cups flour

½ teaspoon salt

½ teaspoon baking powder

1 teaspoon baking soda

1 teaspoon ground cloves

1 teaspoon cinnamon

1 teaspoon nutmeg

½ teaspoon ginger

Beat sugar with oil replacement, then add eggs, one at a time, beating well after each addition. Add in pumpkin. Mix all dry ingredients together, then add into pumpkin mixture. Divide into loaf pans coated with non-stick cooking spray, and bake at 325 degrees for 1 hour. (If you make the bigger loaves, it may take 15 to 30 minutes more). Cool in pans for 10 minutes, then dump out and finish cooling.

Serves: 20

Approximate grams of fat per serving: less than .5

Lemon Bread

This is a sweet bread with a tart topping. Delicious! Serve as a dessert or with brunch.

> *½ cup fat-free sour cream*
> *1 cup sugar*
> *4 egg whites, slightly beaten, or egg substitute to equal 2 eggs*
> *1 ⅔ cup flour*
> *1 teaspoon baking powder*
> *½ teaspoon salt*
> *½ cup skim milk*
> *Grated peel of 1 lemon*

> Topping:
> *Juice of 1 lemon*
> *¼ cup sugar*

Beat sour cream and sugar and then add eggs. Mix flour with baking powder and salt. Alternately add flour mixture and milk to other ingredients while stirring. Mix in lemon peel. Bake in loaf pan coated with nonstick cooking spray at 350 degrees for 1 hour.

After you take the bread from the oven, combine ¼ cup sugar and lemon juice. Pour over loaf while it's still hot.

Serves: 10

Approximate grams of fat per serving: less than .5

Easy Cinnamon Coffee Cake

This was one of the first recipes my son tried on his own. It's easy and fast—great to make for breakfast on a cold morning. Eat this while it's warm! Cover leftovers as they will dry out quickly.

1 cup sugar

2 cups flour

2 teaspoons baking powder

2 tablespoons fat-free sour cream

1 ½ cups skim milk

Topping:

2 tablespoons sugar

2 teaspoons cinnamon

Mix dry ingredients. In a smaller bowl mix sour cream with milk, then stir into the dry ingredients. Pour into a 9- × 9-inch pan that's been coated with nonstick cooking spray. Mix sugar and cinnamon, and sprinkle over the top of the uncooked batter. Bake at 350 degrees for 40 minutes.

Serves: 9

Approximate grams of fat per serving: less than .5

Blueberry Muffins

2 cups flour

½ cup light brown sugar

1 tablespoon baking powder

1 teaspoon baking soda

½ teaspoon nutmeg

1 cup fat-free vanilla yogurt

1 cup skim buttermilk

1 cup fresh or frozen (but thawed) blueberries

Mix dry ingredients and set aside. In a separate bowl mix yogurt, buttermilk, and berries. Stir into dry ingredients until just moistened. Lightly coat muffin tin with nonstick cooking spray or use paper muffin cups. Fill muffin cups about ⅔ full. Bake at 375 degrees for 20 minutes, or until muffin tops are browned.

Serves: 12

Approximate grams of fat per serving: less than .5

DESSERTS

Lemon Cheesecake

Who says you can't have cheesecake? This is delicious served with fresh fruit such as kiwi slices, strawberries, or mandarin orange wedges.

¼ cup low-fat graham cracker crumbs

2 packages (8 ounces) fat-free cream cheese

1 can (14 ounces) fat-free sweetened condensed milk

4 egg whites

Egg substitute to equal 1 egg

⅓ cup lemon juice

2 teaspoons vanilla

¼ cup flour

Coat bottom of an 8-inch springform pan with nonstick cooking spray. Sprinkle graham cracker crumbs over the bottom of the pan. Beat cream cheese until consistency is light. Beat in sweetened condensed milk and mix until smooth. Add egg whites, egg substitute, lemon juice, and vanilla. Beat until creamy. Stir in flour, being careful not to overmix the batter after adding the flour. Pour batter over crumbs, and bake at 300 degrees for 45 to 50 minutes. Cheesecake is done when the center is set. Cool, then refrigerate.

Serves: 10

Approximate grams of fat per serving: less than 1

Soft Molasses Drop Cookies

This is an old family recipe I've adapted to the Low-Fat Lifestyle. The cookies are so moist that they tend to stick to each other when stacked, so place a sheet of waxed paper between layers when you store them.

¼ cup Lighter Bake or ½ cup oil replacement

½ cup molasses

½ cup skim milk

1 teaspoon vinegar

½ cup sugar

2 teaspoons baking soda

2 ½ cups flour

1 teaspoon ginger

1 teaspoon cinnamon

¼ teaspoon nutmeg

½ teaspoon salt

Mix all the wet ingredients in one bowl, and mix the dry ingredients in another bowl. Combine ingredients and beat together until mixed. Bake on cookie sheets lightly coated with nonstick cooking spray at 350 for about 8 to 10 minutes. Cool on a rack.

Yield: approximately 48 cookies

Approximate grams of fat per serving: trace

Individual Hot Fruit Pies

I created these when my family wanted something hot and sweet on a cold night. You can use any flavor of canned pie filling you like. These pies are best served right from the oven with a small scoop of fat-free vanilla ice cream.

6 sheets phyllo dough (find this in the freezer section of your grocery store)
1 can fat-free fruit pie filling (apple, cherry, or blueberry)
Sugar

Place 1 sheet of phyllo dough on your counter, and lightly coat exposed side with nonstick cooking spray. This dough is very thin, so work carefully with it to avoid tearing it.

Spoon about 2 tablespoons of pie filling into the center of the dough. Fold the bottom third of the dough over the filling, then fold the top third down over the inside fold of dough. Fold the dough on the left over the filled area, then roll the filled area toward the right to make what looks like a miniature burrito.

Place the pies on a baking sheet coated with nonstick cooking spray, and lightly spray the tops of the pies with cooking spray. Sprinkle pies with sugar. Bake at 400 degrees for 10 to 15 minutes. The dough should be very crispy. Serve immediately!

Serves: 6

Approximate grams of fat per serving: 1

Lemonade Pie

This is a supereasy, no-bake pie. Cool and light, it's perfect for summer evenings.

1 can fat-free sweetened condensed milk

1 can (6 ounces) frozen lemonade concentrate

1 container (8 ounces) fat-free nondairy whipped topping (such as Cool Whip)

1 reduced-fat prepared graham cracker pie crust (6 ounces)

Gently stir the sweetened condensed milk and lemonade together, then fold in the whipped topping. Spoon mixture into pie shell. Refrigerate for 2 hours before serving. This is also good with fat-free cherry pie filling spooned on top.

Serves: 8

Approximate grams of fat per serving: 3.5

Watermelon and Raspberry Sorbet

One summer I bought two seedless watermelons—one of my favorite summer fruits—and was given another. What to do with all this melon? I whipped up this light and cool dessert and served it to my friends the next day.

1 cup water

⅔ cup sugar

5 cups watermelon chunks, without seeds

4 teaspoons fresh lemon juice

1 cup fresh or frozen raspberries

In a saucepan make a sugar syrup by simmering water with sugar, stirring until sugar dissolves. In a blender, purée watermelon, sugar syrup, lemon juice, and ½ cup raspberries. Strain this mixture through a fine sieve to separate out the raspberry seeds. Chill this until cold—about 2 hours. Freeze this mixture in an ice-cream maker, according to the manufacturer's directions. Serve with the remaining raspberries.

Serves: 6

Approximate grams of fat per serving: less than .5

OTHER GOOD STUFF

Fruit Smoothies

When I have more fruit than we can eat before it spoils, I cut it into chunks, put it into freezer bags, and freeze it until I want to have a fruit smoothie. It's a great way to use leftover fruit salad too!

½ cup frozen chunks of any fruit (apples, pears, peaches, berries,
mango—anything!)

½ cup fat-free yogurt—choose any fruit flavor (it doesn't have to match
the fruit you're adding)

½ cup apple juice or orange juice

Add all ingredients into a blender, and purée until smooth. Add a little more of any ingredient until you get the desired consistency. More frozen fruit will make a thicker drink, and more juice will thin it out.

Serves: 1

Approximate grams of fat per serving: less than 1

Banana Chocolate Milk Shake

1 frozen banana (about 5 frozen chunks)
1 tablespoon fat-free chocolate syrup
1 cup skim milk

Peel your bananas, and break them into bite-size chunks before freezing them.

Add all ingredients to the blender, and purée until smooth. Add more banana chunks for a thicker shake and more milk for a thinner one. Or use strawberry syrup for a strawberry-banana shake.

Serves: 1

Approximate grams of fat per serving: trace

Spinach Dip

For parties, serve this dip in a hollowed-out round of sourdough bread.

1 package (10 ounces) chopped frozen spinach, thawed and well drained
1 cup fat-free mayonnaise
1 cup fat-free sour cream
1 package dried vegetable soup mix
½ cup chopped green onions
1 can water chestnuts, drained and chopped

Mix all ingredients and refrigerate several hours. Serve with chunks of sourdough bread or low-fat crackers.

Serves: a crowd

Approximate grams of fat per serving: trace

Fruit Dip

This light and cool dip is delicious with any kind of fruit. Put a dollop on a bowl of fresh fruit salad, or let your guests spear chunks of fruit on toothpicks and dunk them into a bowl of this refreshing dip.

> *1 package (3 ounces) instant vanilla pudding*
> *1 ½ cups skim milk*
> *½ cup orange juice*
> *1 cup fat-free sour cream*

Mix, dip, eat.

Serves: a crowd

Approximate grams of fat per serving: trace

Onion or Ranch Dip

I've never seen onion soup mix with fat in it, but some of the Ranch dressing packets do contain fat. Read the labels and find one that is fat-free.

> *1 carton fat-free sour cream*
> *1 packet onion soup mix or Ranch dressing mix*

Stir ingredients together and refrigerate for at least 1 hour. Enjoy with veggies or baked chips.

Serves: a crowd

Approximate grams of fat per serving: 0

Salsa

This recipe is refreshing on a hot day! Serve with baked tortilla chips or with your favorite Mexican meal.

4 firm large tomatoes, chopped

½ cup chopped red onion

½ cup chopped cilantro

1 tablespoon jalapeños (more or less to taste)

1 tablespoon lime juice

¼ teaspoon garlic powder

Mix all ingredients and chill about 1 hour before serving.

Serves: at least 1 (I always have to make several batches before I get any!)

Approximate grams of fat per serving: trace

The Low-Fat Soul

What Does It Mean to Have a Low-Fat Soul?

Let us lay aside every weight, and the sin which so easily ensnares us, and let us run with endurance the race that is set before us.

—HEBREWS 12:1 (NKJV)

In Part 1 we talked about living out the Low-Fat Lifestyle in our eating choices and how that affects our physical performance. We learned how to stock our kitchens with low-fat, no-fat, all-flavor options and how to enjoy dining out while not punishing our bodies with high-fat foods. We've even had a chance to try out a number of tasty, easy-to-make, easy-to-enjoy, Low-Fat Lifestyle recipes!

So where do we go next? Into the soul. As I explained in the introduction, the Low-Fat Lifestyle involves not only the physical; it extends to *all* of life—body, soul, and spirit. But before we move into this discussion, let's clarify the meaning of *soul* as we'll use it here.

Many people use the terms *soul* and *spirit* interchangeably—in fact, these words at times mean the same thing in the Bible. But some believe the soul relates more to the mind while the spirit relates more to our relationship with God. These are fine lines and there are numerous scholarly books on this subject (you know, books with unpronounceable words and lots of text written in Hebrew and Greek). We don't want to get into a long theology discussion, so for our purposes we'll keep it simple. Here, *soul* will pertain to that part of us that thinks, dreams, feels, and wills to act—that makes the choices about daily life. Then, in Part 3, we'll allow *spirit* to refer to the part of us that is in relationship with God.

I'll dive into our exploration of how the Low-Fat Lifestyle touches our soul by telling a story.[1]

WEIGHED DOWN

This story begins on the dry, dusty plains of the Valley of Elah. The ground is thirsty, but it will soon be flooded—not with rain but with the blood of desperate, dangerous men. On one side of the valley stands the army of Israel. Camped on a hill and dressed for battle, the fighting forces of King Saul have been waiting—forty days, in fact—for the inevitable battle to come.

Across the valley are the enemy camps of the Philistine warriors, intent on making the Israelite people their slaves. And in between, a giant roars. Goliath, a Philistine from Gath, stands over nine feet tall and is outfitted in armor that weighs more than one hundred pounds. He strikes terror into the hearts of Saul's soldiers.

"Choose someone to fight for you," shouts the giant. "If your man is able to kill me, then we will be your slaves." A wicked grin crosses his face. "But if *I* kill *him,* you will be our slaves!"

Not surprisingly, none of the Israelites volunteer…until finally a young man, David, son of Jesse, steps forward. In the king's tent, Saul tries to prepare David for battle. He places a bronze helmet on the lad's head, wraps a coat of chain mail around his torso, and straps a mighty sword around his waist. David is ready to fight. Or is he?

The young man takes one step, then two, and immediately realizes these accouterments meant to save his life will surely kill him! They are so large and heavy that he can barely move. So he does what must have seemed foolish to those around him at the time but was really the wisest thing he could do. He *simplifies*. He strips down his battle gear to its bare essentials. He unstraps the sword and casts off the armor until he is free to move and attack. Then carrying only what he needs—a slingshot and five smooth stones—he races out to face a giant.

The rest is history. David, of course, felled the oak of a Philistine, and his story remains legendary and awe inspiring to this day.

Have you ever wondered what might have happened if David hadn't taken the time to simplify? What if he had gone out to fight encumbered with heavy nonessentials that weighed him down?

Have you ever wondered why we allow the busyness and cares of this world to weigh down our own lives today? If so, then read on and let's discover together how a Low-Fat Lifestyle can strengthen our souls, allowing us to live lives of simple abundance and gain victory over the giants we battle each day.

SIMPLE ABUNDANCE

Remember the creed of the Low-Fat Lifestyle: *Daily I will fill my life with an abundance of that which is healthy, so that I will no longer need—or eventually even want—that which is unhealthy.*

The same principle applies to the way you feed your soul. Unfortunately, our consumer-obsessed society promotes lifestyle attitudes that are often not in the best interests of your soul. Here are just a few of our culture's prevailing philosophies:

"Get all you can while the getting's good!"
"He who dies with the most toys wins!"
"Money makes the world go 'round!"
"Look out for number one—yourself!"

So we find ourselves going through life at breakneck speed, working ourselves to death trying to acquire everything society tells us we need: a new car (after all, mine is three years old); a new house (hey, interest rates are low); a new wardrobe (I've got to keep up with the latest styles); and a new job (longer hours but better pay).

That kind of stress-filled, soul-sickening lifestyle isn't what God intended for his children. Rather, Christ came to bring us a life of simple abundance where our souls find contentment regardless of our circumstances: "I came to give life—life in all its fullness" (John 10:10, NCV). It's the kind of life the apostle Paul lived and that allowed him to say, "I know what it is to be in need, and I know what it is to have plenty. I have learned the secret of being content in any and every situation, whether well fed or hungry, whether living in plenty or in want" (Philippians 4:12).

It's a state of mind I like to call the low-fat soul. This is an attitude that seeks to clear away the unhealthy emotional and mental clutter of life and fills our souls instead with healthier ways of thinking that yield the fruit of peace, joy, and satisfaction.

Now, let me be clear here. I'm not suggesting that it's wrong to buy a new home or to update your wardrobe. But I *am* suggesting that our consumer-driven culture, which often advocates accumulation and celebrates superficiality, can be taken to an extreme. When this happens, it becomes an unhealthy situation for your soul. Yet instead of suffering from medical illnesses, your soul suffers from emotional sickness such as stress, discontent, frustration, depression, greed, selfishness, arrogance, and so much more.

LESS IS MORE

The low-fat soul, then, is one that shuns the pursuit of "things" and instead chooses to revel in the abundance of the present moment. The person with this kind of attitude seeks to balance the demands of life with the needs of the soul. He or she is someone who, like David of old, knows when to strip away the attachments of the world in order to live more freely and effectively. If it were an equation, it would look like this:

$$Less = More$$

Back in chapter 1 we talked about the positive changes that result from reducing fat in our diets. In that situation, less fatty intake actually equals *more* food—you can eat either a plate full of fat-free foods or a tiny amount of fat-soaked French fries. So cutting out the French fries means you can fill up on baked potatoes instead.

The same principle applies to your soul. When you learn to cut out the "fatty intake" of the mind and heart (consumerism, pursuit of things, investment in the temporary, stress-inducing busyness), you actually gain *more* in the areas that matter to your soul (time, freedom, contentment, joy).

So how do you know what to cut out of—and what to keep in—your soul's diet? As with your eating habits, it starts by honestly assessing your fatty intake.

When I was in college, I briefly lived with a family in which the husband and wife were both addicted to television. For that family, television was a fatty intake they couldn't live without, and it interfered with every other area of their lives.

It started with soap operas, and believe it or not, it was the husband and his college-aged brother who were most captivated by these daytime dramas. From noon until four o'clock every afternoon, they were glued to the television. The husband was self-employed and tried to work around his favorite shows, but eventually they took over so much of his life that he lost his business. This couple's financial troubles added to other stresses in their marriage, and eventually they divorced.

This may seem like an extreme case to you, but it's not. We are often addicted to things that, before we know it, overtake our lives. And while fatty foods are easy to identify, the fat that our souls crave can be difficult for us to spot. Only self-honesty can reveal it to us—or a loving friend who is willing to point it out.

What is the fat in your soul? What inappropriate values, priorities, attitudes, and activities do you need to eliminate to restore your emotional health, refresh your soul, and make room for the fullness of God? Just as we first addressed our eating habits by writing down what we ate, you'll find it extremely helpful to account for your time over the course of a week or two. Start by writing down exactly how you spent your time today (record this in your journal or in a notebook). When did you rise? When did you sleep? How much time did you take for grooming? for household responsibilities? for family activities? chatting with friends? at work? at church? volunteering? watching television? reading?

The point of keeping this log isn't to show how busy or lazy you are. It's just to see how you're presently spending your time and investing your energy. After a week or two, you should have a good idea of what the major time expenditures are in your day. Then you can consider which of these expenditures are valuable to your soul and which are unimportant "fats" in your life.

CHOOSING THE LOW-FAT SOUL

So how will you know what to keep, what to cut out, and what to pursue in your life? In the next three chapters we'll discuss specifically what to keep, cut, and pursue, but for now let me share with you a principle I've found helpful:

It's all about choices.

Life is, in essence, a series of choices—big and small, monumental and mundane. Each attitude and action is like a seed planted in your soul. When that seed matures, you will reap either satisfaction or dissatisfaction in your life. So as you approach the myriad choices you face each day, do your best to choose the attitude or action that will bring about a harvest of peace, contentment, joy, and satisfaction. And avoid "fatty" attitudes and actions that will encumber your soul with unneeded responsibilities, unwanted stress, and time stolen from your family.

The low-fat soul is about choosing meaningful priorities, identifying what brings health to your soul, and then filling yourself to the brim with those parts of life until you don't need—or even want—the second-best things that may have been keeping you from the simple abundance God

has had in store for you all along. My husband, Mike, once wrote a poem
that expresses this concept well:

If in the course of traveling life's road
You find yourself choosing
Between another dollar and the smile of a child,
Choose the smile, for it'll bring happiness long after the dollar
    is gone.

If you encounter a patented program guaranteed to make millions
And a person willing to give a listening ear,
Choose the listening ear, for money is deaf to your sorrows.

If you find a diamond mine filled with gems of great value
And a person who will love you for life,
Choose the lover, and make gemstone memories of your life
    together.

And if you find the choice is between
God and anything else,
Choose God, for then you've chosen eternal life.[2]

Let me recommend a helpful exercise. Find a blank page in your journal or in a notebook, and draw a line down the middle to make two
columns. At the top of the left column write "Five Time Investments That
Bring Me Joy." Label the right column "Five Time Investments That
Drain My Joy."

Take as long as you like to fill in the columns. For instance, in the left column you might list things such as *family* or *best friend* or *camping* or *cooking* or *travel*. You alone know what will go in the columns, but be honest!

When you're done, take time to evaluate your lists. Chances are at least one (possibly all) of the items in the right column are high-fat intakes for your soul. That is, they require your time but don't give health and vitality to your soul in return. The items you list in the left column are likely better, low-fat options for your soul. They require some time investment but return peace, joy, satisfaction, and fulfillment—the kinds of things your soul needs most.

Do you sometimes have that nagging feeling that you want more out of life? I know *I* want more! I want my home life to be low-fat. I want my career to be low-fat. I want my finances to be low-fat. I want all of these to be full of God's goodness. I want my soul to overflow with God's love. The question now is, How can I rearrange my life to allow me to pursue—and benefit from—a low-fat soul?

Let's invest the time to answer this question in practical, productive ways. As we journey together through the areas of our homes, careers, and finances, notice how these aspects of our lives are intertwined. Each affects the other. Our financial health makes a difference in how we approach our careers and our homes. Likewise, the quality of our home life makes a significant impact on our careers and finances. These aspects of life work in synergy with one another, so it's important that each area be low-fat and healthy. And it all starts with the next chapter, so turn the page, and let's go exploring!

SEVEN

The Low-Fat Home Life

Come to me, all you who are weary and burdened, and I
will give you rest.

—MATTHEW 11:28

Tuesday, March 26, 2002, was an unusual night in Ridgewood, New
Jersey. Town sporting events were cancelled. Churches opted not to hold
meetings on this night. Schools declined the opportunity to assign home-
work. It took months of planning, but the people of Ridgewood were taking the night off.

Apparently, some of the leaders of Ridgewood, a town of about thirty
thousand people, decided that life had gotten too hectic. So they organized what they called "Ridgewood Family Night—Ready, Set, Relax!" Most
schools, churches, and other organizations agreed to participate, leaving
families with an evening to spend together eating a meal, watching a movie,
or playing a board game.

While I think this is a wonderful idea, it does say something about
our society and about us as individuals that it would take months of planning and a citywide effort for families in an American town to spend one
evening together. Are we that pressed for time? Are our lives really that

busy? Have we actually forgotten how to take it easy to the point where we need others to force us into a night off?

My guess is that we indeed have. I doubt that any one of us would say things like, "I *want* to have a busy schedule each day. I prefer to be sleep deprived. I choose to have a lot of stress weigh me down. I hope I don't get to relax one minute today." Yet somehow we make choices that ensure these statements come true. How can we turn this around and give ourselves low-fat home lives?

Let's look at this question by dividing our home lives into two areas: the household and the home. The *household* will include the physical property where we live and the tasks required to keep this place functioning. The *home* will focus on the people who live in that household and others who regularly spend time there. (Even if you're single or living alone, family and friends help to create your home.)

THE LOW-FAT HOUSEHOLD

The book of Luke tells of a man who wanted his brother to share the family inheritance with him. This man came to Jesus and requested that Jesus tell the wealthy brother how to divide the money. Jesus declined this opportunity, then he said to those present, "Watch out! Be on your guard against all kinds of greed; a man's life does not consist in the abundance of his possessions" (Luke 12:15).

Then Jesus told the people a story:

The ground of a certain rich man produced a good crop. He thought to himself, "What shall I do? I have no place to store my crops."

Then he said, "This is what I'll do. I will tear down my barns and build bigger ones, and there I will store all my grain and my goods. And I'll say to myself, 'You have plenty of good things laid up for many years. Take life easy; eat, drink and be merry.'"

But God said to him, "You fool! This very night your life will be demanded from you. Then who will get what you have prepared for yourself?" (Luke 12:16-20)

Jesus concluded this story with a warning: "This is how it will be with anyone who stores up things for himself but is not rich toward God" (verse 21).

This story has a wonderful application for us as we try to live the Low-Fat Lifestyle, especially as we create low-fat households. It is not what we have that's important; rather, it is our relationships with God, family, and friends that deserve top priority.

The man in Jesus' story had more than he could use. We can look at him and say, "Why didn't he give some away? He could have fed hungry people instead of hoarding his wealth." We see that greed and gathering were forms of fat in this man's life. And while he imagined that his wealth would allow him to relax and enjoy life, it's highly possible that his stress skyrocketed as he had to consider how to manage and protect his holdings. After all, barns had to be built and maintained. What about robbers who might steal that grain? What about hired help to oversee the operation? And so it goes. An abundance of things can lead to greed, stress, worries, and other fats that we'd like to live without. So let's start there—with the stuff, the clutter—that fattens our souls.

Cut the Clutter

I have to admit I'm someone who often dreams of having a bigger home. I imagine spacious rooms, wide hallways, and more cabinets than I can fill. I could entertain crowds—or at least host our Bible study group. I could do aerobics in the privacy of my own home without knocking my knees on the furniture. I would finally have a place to put all my stuff. Ah, the dream of it all!

What's interesting to me, though, is that when we first moved into our current house many years ago, we thought we'd never be able to fill all the space. Several rooms were left empty for months because we didn't have enough furniture. I didn't know what I'd do with all the cabinets and shelves. After years of living in apartments with tiny cement patios, our yard seemed huge. But now, after ten years in this house, it sometimes feels cramped to me.

As Mike and I were talking about our home (and my dreams of a bigger one), I realized the primary problem was having too many things in too small a space. We'd accumulated a lot of stuff over the years, making our house seem smaller. It was time to trim some fat from our household to make room for the living beings within.

Mike wondered aloud one day if we could find ten items in each room that we didn't need and could part with immediately. I was willing to give it a try, so we started our hunt. The bedrooms were no trouble at all: clothes we hadn't worn in years, books that were outdated or no longer of interest, junk we'd stacked in corners, and magazines that somehow had ended up under the bed. Out they went, either to a secondhand store or the garbage.

Next, we tackled the living room and playroom. Toys missing pieces were tossed, as were more dusty and ancient magazines (under the couch this time). In the kitchen, I found gadgets and gizmos that I wasn't even sure how to use, napkins with pictures of footballs on them that I was saving for a Super Bowl party (never mind that I'd had these napkins for three years and, after three parties, had still never used them), and cookbooks that I know I'll never use (*The Cheese Cookbook* was the first to go). We had started by looking for ten items in each room and easily found fifteen or more. How nice to see the floor again! While I still wouldn't mind having a larger house, I found that having less stuff keeps me from feeling squeezed into the one I've got.

Clutter is a fat we can do without in our households. Yet it's as easy to pile up stacks of stuff as it is to pile a mound of sour cream on a baked potato. And just as some people hire personal cooks and trainers to help them manage their eating and exercise habits, others hire personal organizers who help them manage their households and find places for all their belongings. However, I don't want to pay someone else to get my house in order, and my guess is that you don't either. So instead of hiring professionals, let's implement some helpful strategies to cut the clutter.

Do a "spring" cleaning any time of year. Although spring is the traditional time to clear out the dust and clutter that's accumulated over the year, you can do it anytime. And if the idea of cleaning the whole house or apartment seems daunting, start with one room and go from there. Look for items you don't use anymore, clothing that's out of style or no longer fits, and things that are broken (and that you're willing to admit you're never going to fix). Even though some items are worth keeping for their sentimental value, there's a point when it's time to let a few of these "treasures" go.

Can you find ten expendable items in each room of your house or apartment? Hold a garage sale, take a trip to the dump, or call a local agency like Goodwill or the Salvation Army to have the items removed from your house. Then look at all the space you've got! Like the man in Jesus' parable, we could be giving away from our wealth of things instead of hoarding them for ourselves.

Resist the urge to buy more. I laughed at Mike one Sunday as he was paging through all the newspaper advertisements. "Is there something you need?" I asked, wondering if he hoped to find a pair of shorts on sale.

Mike gave me a sheepish look as he answered, "No, I'm just looking to see what I *might* need."

I knew exactly what he meant. In fact, I'll admit that Mike has had to help me learn to stop buying things that I'll never use, simply because they're on sale.

"This shirt is only one dollar!" I exclaim as I browse through a store.

"It's also an ugly color, you don't have anything that matches it, and it's not your size," Mike comments.

"But it's only *one dollar!*" I repeat. "It's a bargain!"

After purchasing a few of these "bargains" and having them hang in my closet for years until I finally give them away, I've learned that something you don't need is not a bargain, no matter how low the price.

Sure, that vegetable slicer-dicer-chopper combo is a good buy, but will you use it more than once? Is this an item that will take up a lot of space and eventually become clutter? Does it require a lot of cleaning or upkeep? Stop and evaluate your needs before making your purchase.

Value what you have. Just about every time I help Tony clean his room (you know, the annual excavation of closets and dresser drawers), he finds something he forgot he had. "Oh, I remember this!" he exclaims, then plays with this toy for the rest of the day. It can be the same with us. We have so many things that we forget what we have! Why not take inventory and find those useful things you've forgotten about?

When was the last time you got out the family photo albums or those old yearbooks and looked through them? They've been sitting on your shelf for years. Get them out and revel in the memories, sharing them with those you love.

What about the treasured gifts people have given you that you've tucked away as too precious to use? Get them out and use them. Share them. Show them off. What good is a gift that's hidden away?

Once we've cleared away the clutter, we can step back and see what we treasure and want to keep. These are the things that help bring fullness to our hearts, remind us of hard times we've weathered and laughter we've shared, and help us appreciate what others have passed on to us. Keep these things visible in your household instead of the junk and clutter.

Tame the Tasks

Trying to manage all the stuff in our lives creates another fat that I know many of us would like to live without: tasks. These are the chores that are required to keep that household running. The shopping, the laundry, the cooking, the yard work, the maintenance—the list goes on and on.

The tricky part about eliminating tasks is that many of these jobs truly do need to be done. How can we determine which ones aren't that important? How can we get the important tasks done without taking up too much time and adding stress? Here are a few ideas.

Quit being a perfectionist. I've always been someone who takes pride in making foods from scratch. I never used boxed mixes or took shortcuts when cooking. Everything had to be made from step one by my own hands. I enjoyed the praise of family and friends as they ate breads, cookies, casseroles, and other dishes I'd prepared. Then my life changed when I went to work full time. Instead of kneading dough in the afternoon, I was editing manuscripts. Instead of dicing vegetables and grating lemon peels, I was talking to authors. And my family and friends were waiting there, hungry, when I walked through the door at 5:15 each evening.

I tried for a short time (a very short time) to keep up my high standards for cooking. But I finally had to admit I couldn't do it all to my own expectations. I couldn't be a perfectionist cook and still enjoy my life. So I started buying premade salads from delis. I found vegetables that were already sliced and diced. I opted for frozen instead of fresh. Amazingly, life went on and none of us starved.

What tasks could you ease up on? Perhaps you're the kind who wants the entire house to be clean and dusted to perfection. Or you want the yard to be full of flowers and without a weed. Or you iron every piece of laundry. Choose what's important for your high standards and then let some of the other things go. In my case, I still can cook with my perfectionist *low-fat* standards, but not to my perfectionist *homemade* standards.

Eliminate optional tasks. A few years ago, we decided to stop sending out Christmas cards. Even though we could have printed out the address labels on the computer, photocopied a letter, and sent out a generic greeting, we decided it was one task we could cut from our life. We still keep in touch with our family and friends, but we no longer try to keep up with a time-consuming tradition.

This is just one example of the tasks we often *choose* to do that aren't essential. Seeing things on paper helps, so find a blank page in your journal or notebook, and write down your daily, weekly, monthly, and annual tasks. Be as specific as you can.

When you're done, slowly and thoughtfully read over this list. Put a star next to those tasks that are crucial, and either cross off or simplify those that aren't. For example, you might decide that you could cut out regular shopping for gifts and standing in lines at the post office by sending your nieces and nephews money for their birthdays instead of clothing or toys.

Get help. Wouldn't it be great to have a maid, a gardener, and a nanny? Most of us can't afford to regularly pay someone to care for all of our tasks. But if tasks have become overwhelming for you and you can afford to pay someone to help (even occasionally), do it! Let someone else mow your lawn or clean your bathrooms. Even having someone do *a few* of your tasks might cut down on the stress you feel and the load you bear.

Another way to get help is to ask your family. As a mother, I know how tempting it is to do everything for everyone. I've seen friends take complete care of their children and spouses and then when these women need to be away for a night or two, the family is helpless.

I've gotten help with tasks in our home by letting family members get involved with their own care. When Tony was in the second grade, he started packing his own lunches. The following year he started doing his own laundry. He doesn't always pack foods I would eat, and his clothes are sometimes wrinkled, but he's fed and clothed and I don't have to do it for him. Now that he's in junior high school, part of his responsibilities includes preparing one meal for the family each week and cleaning the kitchen afterward.

One caveat about assigning tasks to family members: Don't hold everyone to your standards. If pants aren't pressed with a military-style crease, so what? If there are a couple of leaves on the lawn after your child rakes, muffle any criticism and instead praise the family member for his or her contribution to the household.

Slow Down and Simplify

Remember the old saying, "Stop and smell the roses"? Well, when was the last time you did that? Being in a hurry to get things done adds stress to our lives. As you face the daily responsibilities of managing your household, slow down. Take time to breathe and let those around you do the same.

So often we get stressed out because we didn't choose the shortest line at the grocery store. Next time, determine not to get agitated and instead use the time to pray or chat with the person next to you. You might even let someone else go ahead of you! And the next time you're sitting at a red light, feeling your impatience escalate, take a deep breath, turn up the radio, and enjoy a moment of repose. All your stress isn't going to make that light turn green any faster.

THE LOW-FAT HOME

When I speak to women's groups, I like to do an experiment with them. Would you like to try it yourself? Grab a pencil and a piece of paper. Now draw the face of a penny (don't peek at a real one for help).

After you've done your best artwork, dig under the couch cushions and find a penny to compare with your drawing. How'd you do? Did you get Lincoln facing in the right direction? Did you remember all the words and numbers and put them in the right places? If you're like most of the women I try this with, you can remember a few of the details, but not all of them.

Think about how many times you've held a penny in your hand. You've probably been touching and looking at pennies for years and years, yet you couldn't draw one accurately. This phenomenon is called being "home blind." We've seen the things closest to us for so long and with such regularity that we stop truly looking. We just give a glance and think we know what's there. But it's likely that we've stopped knowing.

Obviously, this phenomenon is most common in our homes. We think we know our family members because we're around them all the time. And perhaps we really did know them at one time and still know the general features that define our families. Yet we might not really *know* them anymore. We might be letting the fat in our homes hinder the depth and quality of our family relationships.

This reminds me of a story about a powerful businessman who was retiring. He knew that many people wanted his job, so at his last company gathering he explained how any eager executive could get his job: "Last week my daughter was married, and as she walked down the aisle, I realized I did not know the name of her best friend, or the last book she read, or her favorite color. That's the price I paid for this job. If you want to pay that price, you can have it."[1]

Compare the sad reflections of this man to a comment made by Dr. James Dobson:

> When all is said and done and the books are closing on your life, I believe your treasures will lie close to home. Your most precious memories will focus on those you loved, those who loved you, and what you did together in the service of the Lord. Those are the basics. Nothing else will survive the scrutiny of time.[2]

The important businessman didn't enjoy the blessings of a low-fat home. He filled up on the tempting fats that edge into our home life and keep us from enjoying the richness of our families, then he realized too late the truth of Dr. Dobson's insight. These fats seem so appealing at the time, but just as fatty foods clog our arteries, fatty activities and attitudes clog our relationships.

What makes a low-fat home? Remember our creed: *Daily I will fill my life with an abundance of that which is healthy, so that I will no longer need—or eventually even want—that which is unhealthy.* In our homes, this means an abundance of family, friends, and free time as well as the intentional avoidance of fats that may keep us from enjoying these vital priorities.

Family: "Come Enjoy Us"

When Tony was about four, he and Mike were getting ready to play a game. Tony came into the kitchen where I was busy washing dishes to ask me to join them. However, Tony's words got tangled as he spoke, and he instead said, "Mom, do you want to come *enjoy* us?" I smiled at these words at the time, and ever since, our family has repeated them as an invitation.

Do you want to come enjoy us? To me this means much more than what Tony actually said. It means "Do you want to spend time with us? Do you want to show that you love us more than a clean home or a job or a position at the church?"

What are the fats to which you may be home blind? What priorities or preoccupations keep you from enjoying your family? Many fats keep us from our families, but my guess is that the most "fat grams" in our home lives come from activities: sports, clubs, music lessons, choirs, church activities, school programs.

We want our children and ourselves to be well-rounded members of society. We want our children to have advantages we didn't have, to make friends and be physically active. Yet there's got to be a limit. One woman

I know told me her family has one hour on Wednesdays that they can spend together. *One hour!* The rest of their week they spend apart from one another, engaged in various activities. I'm sure many of the pursuits are worthwhile—but at the expense of family time? Remember, it's all about choices.

My parents gave our family a wonderful example of making good choices. When I was about ten, I wanted to join a Christian organization similar to the Girl Scouts. My parents had nothing against this organization, yet they also knew how important it was for family members, especially parents and children, to spend time together. My parents gave me an option: "You can join this club, or you can spend every Tuesday evening this year with your mom."

I chose the time with my mom. With five kids in my family, a whole evening with Mom each week was a real treat! We walked around malls, did sewing projects, stopped for a donut or ice cream (this was before I knew anything about fat), and tried out new recipes. Many of our outings cost no money. All of them cost time. And all of them filled my soul with a sense of safety, the knowledge of my mother's love (and Dad's, too, since he was hanging out with the other four kids), and an opportunity to know Mom better.

Consider your own family's activities. What are the fats that keep you from making the best choices for their life and health? How can you set limits on the number and types of activities? How will setting limits help each person? And then, what *are* the best, soul-nourishing activities?

As a family, brainstorm the activities that would bring you all closer together and would nuture the growth of healthy souls. Choose these life-giving activities, and leave the fatty ones behind.

A True Friend Is a Treasure

We love to hear stories of true friends. Consider the popular movies of recent years that involve two or more people thrown together by various circumstances. There was the crazy-yet-caring group of women in *Steel Magnolias* and the liberating friendship between "Red" and Andy in *The Shawshank Redemption*. The connection between Miss Daisy and her chauffer, Hoke, in *Driving Miss Daisy*. The hijinks of detectives Martin Riggs and Roger Murtaugh in the *Lethal Weapon* movies. The boys who shoot for the stars in *October Sky*. Even toys, monsters, and storybook characters in movies such as *Toy Story, Monster's, Inc.,* and *Shrek* remind us of the importance of true friends.

What are your friendships like? Enduring friendships give us strength and courage in tough times and help us laugh no matter what's going on. True friends fill our lives with health and happiness.

Friendship, of course, is a two-way street. Many of us had mothers who told us that to *have* a friend you have to *be* a friend. This means reaching out to others with kindness, providing a listening ear, going the extra mile, and extending forgiveness. So when it comes to quality friend-ships, we must first consider what kind of friend we are to others. How do your friends perceive you? Are you gracious and kind or snappy and demanding? Do you fill the lives of those around you with health or harm? How could you be a better friend?

Next, take a look at the friends who fill your life. Which of these people enrich your life, help you grow, and foster vitality? Which ones seem to drain your soul and drag you down?

It sounds cruel to say that we should consider cutting some friends from our lives. After all, there are times when friends are down and need our help and encouragement. When it comes to friendship, our goal first and foremost should be to demonstrate devotion, commitment, and loyalty. But let's also remember that we're making choices for a healthy lifestyle, and it is sometimes the case that a friendship stagnates or becomes one-sided, an emotional drain.

Many years ago I became friends with a woman I'll call Yolanda. Our husbands worked together, and our kids were close in age. I would call Yolanda regularly and set up times to get together. She often didn't have time to meet or would cancel at the last minute. After this happened several times, I began to feel as though our relationship wasn't important. I realized that I was always the one initiating our get-togethers. So I decided to stop calling Yolanda and see how long it would be before she called me. One week went by, then two, then a month, then two. It hurt for a while, but I realized that I was putting a lot into trying to make a friendship work when it simply *wasn't* working. I have no hard feelings toward Yolanda; I just realize that developing a friendship with me wasn't a priority for her. What's more, it was becoming a drain for me, a fat I could live without.

Over the years I've had other opportunities to consider the time I'm putting into various friendships. I may not see some friends for several years, yet I still feel close to them and would do whatever I could to help them in a crisis. With other friends, I've realized that I was blessed with a season of their friendship, and that season eventually passed. Trying to hold on to friendships that are "out of season" can be draining.

On the other hand, I think of the friendships that bring me fullness and strength. These are the friendships I want to cultivate and grow. I *choose* to make them a priority for my soul health. I have three dear friends whom I regularly meet for lunch. While we eat our sandwiches and watch our kids play outside, we talk about the deeper issues in our lives. We care for each other, confront each other, pray for each other, and love each other. Choosing the friendships of these women has brought me joy and strength and has helped me grow in different areas of my life.

Consider evaluating your friendships to determine which ones are helping you grow and which ones may be merely siphoning off your time and energy. Then plan how you can spend more time with those friends who bring health into your life and less time with those who add fat.

The High Cost of Free Time

A friend I'll call Cathy shared with me that she was undergoing a lot of stress—so much stress that she had become depressed and didn't know how to handle this change in her emotions. Cathy sought help from a counselor who assisted her in sorting through the events and activities of her life.

At one point, the counselor asked Cathy, "What do you do for your own enjoyment? What activities are you involved in simply because they bring you joy and pleasure?"

Cathy couldn't think of anything.

She told me,

My husband would think nothing of coming home from church on a Sunday and watching several hours of football because that's what he wanted to do. I didn't have a problem with my husband doing this, but I would never come home from church and say, "I rented a movie for myself to watch this afternoon," then go ahead and watch it. I didn't feel that I had the right to enjoy myself like that. I would have felt guilty thinking only of myself.

I can relate to Cathy's situation. After spending time at work, with my family, at church, and volunteering in a few activities, I don't have much free time. And when I do have free time, I feel guilty about doing things just for myself. Shouldn't I be working in the yard? Shouldn't I be helping my son with his book report? Shouldn't I be doing something *constructive* with my time?

Who says *relaxing* isn't constructive? Not taking time for ourselves can make our lives more stressful, and stress is definitely a fat we can live without. Consider these facts:

- Forty-three percent of adults suffer adverse health effects due to stress.
- One million Americans miss work each day due to stress.
- Seventy-five to 90 percent of doctor visits are for stress-related complaints.[3]

Stress can lead to a variety of physical ailments as well as anxiety, exhaustion, and depression. Simply facing the day-to-day demands of our careers, finances, families, and homes can be overwhelming. We begin to feel as if our candle is burning at both ends—or has already burned out!

We must allow ourselves a healthful amount of free time. What could this look like in your life? Think about these ideas:

- Take a walk alone or with a friend.
- Rent a movie you've wanted to see for a long time.
- Lie in the hammock or on a blanket under a shade tree.
- Curl up with a book.
- Take a long hot bath, complete with bath oils and candles.
- Stretch out on the couch while listening to your favorite CD.
- Read the whole newspaper.

- Try something new. Explore. Be curious.
- Put the kids to bed, then sit outside and count the stars.

How can you find the time for such leisure activities? You plan time for other people and other things, so start planning time for *you*. When someone calls to see if you're free to do something that you're not all that thrilled about doing, it's not dishonest to say, "Thanks, but I've got other plans that evening." Without elaborating, you've said no to a fat and yes to time for yourself. I've literally locked myself in the bathroom for a half-hour to get a bit of time alone. Mike and I have always held to an early bedtime for Tony so that we have time for ourselves at the end of the day.

Entire books have been written on these concepts that help us have a low-fat home life. You'll find some listed in the recommended resources at the end of this book. For now, focus on what's important in your home. Cut away what isn't. The choice is yours. Choose the best.

EIGHT

The Low-Fat Career

> He has showed you, O man, what is good. And what does
> the LORD require of you? To act justly and to love mercy
> and to walk humbly with your God.
>
> —MICAH 6:8

This past Christmas season, my friend Heidi was lamenting the fact that she had to attend a company party with her husband, who is an attorney. Heidi thought no one would be interested in making conversation with her since she's a stay-at-home mom who homeschools their daughters.

"All the snooty business types just ignore me or roll their eyes when they find out what I do all day," she complained. "It's going to be a long, boring evening."

I joked with Heidi, telling her she should invent a wildly unusual career for the evening. "You could tell people you're a sky-diving instructor," I suggested. "Or that you sculpt gargoyles for the homes of the rich and famous. Then you can pretend to be snooty right back since your career would be much more interesting than any of theirs."

We laughed, and Heidi later survived the party (going as herself instead of an undercover spy or trapeze artist). But the truth of Heidi's situation is just one of many issues related to having a career—especially for women:

- What if my career isn't glamorous or important enough? Will others lose respect for me?
- Should I be a stay-at-home mom or a work-outside-the-home mom?
- What if my career is unfulfilling?
- How do I cope when my career leaves me feeling drained and without time for my family or anything else?

I'll be honest and tell you I'm right in the middle of these issues. I'm not Moses preaching from the mountaintop to the crowd below. I'm standing at the foot of the mountain with everyone else, trying to apply the words of wisdom I'm hearing. I do know that many words of wisdom about the Low-Fat Lifestyle apply to my career, and I'm doing my best to implement them in my life. I'd like to share with you what I know to be true, and together we can work toward putting these principles into practice.

WHAT'S MY CAREER?

First, let me address those of you who might be saying, "I don't have a career." You may be a parent who doesn't consider what you do a career (even though parenting is the most important work you'll ever do). You might be working a job that seems like a dead-end position and hoping this doesn't become your career. Or you might be unemployed. It doesn't matter. You have a career. Let me give you an example from the life of my friend Jana.

Every Tuesday through Saturday, Jana gets up early and heads to the post office. There she sorts through mail and puts bundles and packages into various bins and containers. Then she loads it all into her white Jeep—the kind in which the steering wheel is on the right side instead of the left. Finally she drives away from town to her rural route. Jana is, of course, a mail carrier, but as for her *career*…well, that's a different story.

Jana is a world-class pray-er. She talks to God all day long, reminding him of her coworkers and each person along her route. She occasionally takes time to visit with the elderly and lonely people who meet her at their mailboxes. She may be the only friendly face those people see that day. She listens to what God tells her about these people and offers words of guidance and support. And then she prays for these people some more. When she's not driving her route, Jana loves to dig into the Scriptures for words of encouragement or guidance to share with family or friends.

Mike and I love to have Jana pray for us. In fact, when Mike was very sick, and the doctors didn't know what was wrong, I would lay awake at night praying to God that he would wake up Jana and remind her to pray for Mike!

While Jana is paid to deliver mail, I believe her real career is that of a prayer warrior. If she went to a party like the one Heidi attended and introduced herself saying, "Hi! I'm Jana. I'm a prayer warrior," she would get more strange looks than if she told people she was a CIA operative. But it would be true!

For some of us, it's easy to identify our careers. You might simply say, "I'm a teacher…a scientist…a librarian…a mother." Others might need to think more carefully to identify what their career is. If you're not employed in the traditional sense of the word, you may find that your volunteer activities are your career, or your time spent with others, or any other activities that take up large portions of your time.

You do have a career, and it's up to you to make sure it's a healthy part of your life that is low on fat and high on joy. I doubt any of us want a career that's bad for our health, so let's explore what we should nurture and what we can trim in our careers.

GETTING OUR PRIORITIES STRAIGHT

In previous chapters we've discovered that most of the Low-Fat Lifestyle comes down to making choices. The word I'd like us to focus on as we consider career choices is *priorities*. "What are my priorities, and how do they help me have a low-fat career?"

I've seen a simple science experiment many times in my life that wonderfully demonstrates the importance of getting our priorities in order. First, I fill a jar with stones. I could use walnuts, marbles, or something else of equivalent size. My jar looks full, but I notice spaces between these items. So I take a few handfuls of dry rice (or sand) and pour it into the jar. This fills all the cracks and empty spaces. Now the jar is full. (Well, I could still pour some water in there, since there are tiny spaces between the grains of rice—but the stones and rice will do.)

I pour out all of this onto the counter and separate the stones from the rice. Now I put the same amount of rice back into the jar and, of course, there's still room left. So I start to put the stones back in on top of the rice. I'm using exactly the same amount of rice and the same stones, but now the stones won't fit. I can cram only a few stones in before the jar is filled.

This experiment is a beautiful illustration of the importance of our priorities. We have to put the most important pieces, the biggest pieces, into our lives first. Then we can add the smaller things, the things that are less important. We have to get our priorities straight so we won't feel as if we're cramming in stones that won't fit.

How do we determine our priorities? We know that there are some things we must have in our lives, and then there are other things that can fill in the gaps. But how do we tell the difference between the important, healthful things that fill us with joy and the less-important, fatty things that we should use only to fill in the gaps—or leave out entirely? Keep in mind our creed: *Daily I will fill my life with an abundance of that which is healthy, so that I will no longer need—or eventually even want—that which is unhealthy.* How does this apply to priorities and careers? Let's break it down into three areas so we can better understand our priorities: purpose, passion, and people.

THE POWER OF PURPOSE

What's the purpose of your career? Does your answer sound like one of these?

- To earn a living
- To serve God
- To help my family find happiness
- To keep my household functioning efficiently
- To get ahead in life
- To pass on what I know

You might feel that your purpose is obvious—or you might not have a clue as to what purpose your career serves. The purpose of your career doesn't have to be the purpose of your whole life, but they're usually intertwined. Again, we can find guidance in the ancient wisdom of the Bible.

Our General Purpose

Micah 6:8, quoted at the beginning of this chapter, reminds us of God's desire for his children: to act justly, to love mercy, and to walk humbly with him. In the eyes of our Creator, these are foundational to everything else we do in life. These goals also serve as a good place to begin evaluating our work. Does your career give you opportunities to act justly? to demonstrate mercy? to show humility? to express your faith in God?

You might think, *I'd have to have a career like Mother Teresa for these purposes to be evident!* Not really. If your career allows you to live ethically, to show kindness and compassion, and to humbly express your faith, it might just be God's path for you. (And note that word *humbly*. There's something to be said for living a quiet faith instead of loudly and obnoxiously proclaiming the name of Jesus—but that's another topic altogether!) Let Micah 6:8 be the foundational purpose for your career.

Our Gifted Purpose

We also know that God has a purpose for each of us because he's given his children gifts—spiritual gifts. These are listed in several places in the Bible. (For starters read Romans 12:6-8; 1 Corinthians 12:4-11; Ephesians 4:11-13; and 1 Peter 4:10-11.) And what's the point of receiving a gift that you never use? If I treat my gifts from God the way I treat the frumpy nightgown that a well-meaning (and unnamed) someone gave me for Christmas, then what's the point of having them?

The point is this: Look for ways in which your career allows you to use your spiritual gifts. Think again of my friend Jana. It's not a part of her mail-carrier job description to pray for people along her route, but her job doesn't stop her from doing this either. She has a gift, and it's important that she be able to use it in her career as a prayer warrior.

If you're not sure what your spiritual gifts are, talk to your pastor or check a Christian bookstore for resources to help you discern the particular strengths God has given you.

Our Governing Purpose

I'm involved in children's ministry in our church. Many years ago my fellow workers and I decided that we couldn't lead the children well if we didn't have a clear purpose. So a number of us gathered over a period of several weeks and came up with a governing purpose statement we could use to guide our ministry. Whenever someone comes up with a new idea or wants to lead the children in a special activity, we review our purpose statement and ask, "Will this activity, idea, or technique help us achieve our purpose?"

Many ministries and businesses use a governing purpose statement (often called a mission statement). This serves as a guide or a measuring stick against which to test the direction of the business. Likewise, many people have found that a clearly defined mission statement for their personal lives helps them stay focused on the important things while steering clear of life's many distractions.

I'd like to suggest that each of us create a governing purpose statement as it relates to our careers. This statement can help us say yes or no to the various options that come along in our careers, helping us choose where to cut the fat and where to focus our energies.

It may take you some time to consider what you'd like your career purpose statement to say. And remember, it doesn't have to stay the same forever; you can change it over time as you grow into a healthier person. Begin by embracing the general purpose from Micah 6:8 and then get more specific as you consider your spiritual gifts, your interests, the direction you'd like your life to take, the things God has put on your heart to accomplish. Use all of these to shape your career purpose statement.

How will this help you trim the fat from your career? Once you have a clear statement of career purpose, you can use it as a guide. For example, the career purpose statement for a mother might be: "To love and train my children so they will grow into men and women who honor and serve God." Then when life's various activities, commitments, and opportunities come knocking, this mother can test them against her statement. Will the proposed opportunity help her to achieve her purpose or distract her from it? Should she commit or not?

My personal career statement is one word: *balance*. When I'm asked to write, speak, or do other things related to my career, I can ask myself, "Will this opportunity help me maintain balance in my life, or will it throw my life off kilter? Does it compromise my ethics? Does it allow me to work in areas where I'm gifted? Is it a realistic time commitment?" If I do things that compromise my faith, are beyond my abilities, or consume too much time, my life becomes unbalanced. But if I accept projects that help maintain balance in my life and turn down those that don't, I find joy and fulfillment. My career statement serves as a guide for deciding what would add fat to my life and what would promote good health.

Take time now to jot down in a journal or notebook some ideas for your career purpose statement. Start with Micah 6:8. Consider your spiritual gifts. Then personalize it all. What statement will help you trim fat and choose the best? Over the next few days, refine this statement until you're comfortable with it. Then print it out and post it in a place where you will see it every day.

WHAT'S YOUR PASSION?

My friends and family members know how much I love amusement parks, especially Disneyland. Now there's something I feel passionate about! I'll leave the Rocky Mountains any day for Space Mountain or Splash Mountain. What an adrenaline rush! Knowing this, you can imagine how excited I was about being hired to work at an amusement park right out of college (even back then I had roller-coaster fever). I was to work in the human resources department, and Mike and I would get free admission to the park anytime it was open. I couldn't wait for my first day on the job!

I quickly learned that even in an amusement park, life isn't all fun and games. Along with meaningful work (and quick rides on the roller coasters during my lunch breaks), there were also a lot of boring tasks to be done. Fortunately, there was a good balance between the thrills and the tedium, so I usually enjoyed my job. But in reality, it was never something I felt passionate about.

Do you know anyone who *loves* his or her job? Have you ever known someone who couldn't wait to get to work in the morning? Most of us don't characterize our careers in this way. Why not? Even though we usually get to choose our careers, many people feel dissatisfied, bored, frustrated, and stressed about their careers. Those emotions are fats we could all live without!

Passion for our careers is important. Obviously, we'd love to be involved in careers that offer excitement and boost our enthusiasm. Yet even in the most delightful job, there's likely to be some drudgery. Getting the following elements into perspective will help us make choices that keep our careers low-fat and healthy.

Delight

Take a moment to identify the things you love about your career. Maybe you get to help people or make important decisions or use your creative abilities. Write down the three things you find most rewarding about your work.

As you look at your list, take time to thank God for giving you these delights. The next time you're having a rough day at work, remind yourself of the things you enjoy about your job. Make these delights priorities in your career. Whenever possible, focus on putting these aspects first. The more you enjoy your career, the less you're going to feel stressed and angry about what you do each day. Emphasize the abundance and cut the fat.

Drudgery

Numerous people have said to me, "It must be exciting being a writer!" I usually smile and thank them for their interest in what I do. However, occasionally I feel bold and honest enough to respond, "Actually, I sit in an office by myself staring at a computer screen for hours on end, which isn't all that exciting." As much as I love sharing my passions through books and articles, the actual process of writing can be slow and lonely— and I'm a social person who likes to be around others. So while writing is not drudgery, it's not always pure delight either.

The fact is, some things about our careers aren't exciting. And to top it off, many of these things are priorities. Filing? Counting inventory? Sitting through long classes or meetings? All of these may be part of your job. They have to be done. I'm sure you can think of several things about your career that are boring or tedious yet are part of what you get paid to do.

"But wait!" you might say. "I thought pursuing a Low-Fat Lifestyle would allow me to reduce or eliminate drudgery! After all, drudgery is draining, stressful, and often leads to procrastination." Again, it's a choice we make. We may not always be able to reduce or eliminate drugery, but we *can* choose to make the dull tasks enjoyable rather than choosing to complain and procrastinate.

For example, I have a friend named Jeff who worked for many years as a night security guard. Sounds like a boring job, just sitting at a desk for eight hours in a dark building. While the job wasn't exciting by any means, Jeff was allowed to read or write while on duty. So he began writing, and before long he had completed several novels. Jeff isn't a security guard anymore. By making positive choices about his attitudes and actions amid the drudgery of his security guard job, he was able to move into a different career as a writer.

I've heard of people who make games out of the dull parts of their day, who give themselves rewards for getting the tedious tasks done quickly, or who make it a point to look at the bright side of every dark moment. So when I'm feeling lonely in my quiet office, I can think, *Hey, how many people can go to work in their pajamas? I've got it made!* We can find delight even in the dullness.

How about you? Take a moment to identify three aspects of your career that you consider drudgery. Now consider how your attitudes and approach to these tasks might make them more fulfilling. How can your choices about these responsibilities help you find delight?

PEOPLE ARE THE PRIORITY

One of Mike's college professors, Dr. Michael Anthony, often made a comment in his lectures that has stuck with both Mike and me over the years: "Only people count." Dr. Anthony wasn't saying, of course, that

God or other life essentials didn't matter. He used this phrase in the context of ministry and careers. When we get caught up in the programs, the processes, or our performances, we forget what it's all about: people. Only people count!

Jesus provides the best example of this truth. What was Jesus' career? When you boil it all down, Jesus came to earth so that people could know God. Through his life, we could know God. Through his death, we could know God. It was all about people. Even before Jesus, God's intent has always been for people to know him. From the very beginning, through all the trials and wars and good times and bad times, all God has wanted is to draw people to himself. To God, only people count.

Thus, people should be the top priority in our careers. They should be the biggest "stone" in our jars—the stone that is never removed because it's so important.

Some people have careers that allow them to interact with people directly—nurses, teachers, cashiers, social workers. However, just because one's career affords face-to-face communication with people doesn't necessarily mean that he or she is communicating love. All of us can think of a mean teacher or an aloof medical professional. But, fortunately, we can also think of plenty of people who *did* care and make us feel valued. If your career allows you to touch people directly, you have the privilege of using that opportunity fully to demonstrate God's love.

I told you earlier that I'm involved in children's ministry. Every Sunday when I arrive at church, I hope the kids will get something out of the lesson. I hope the teaching time goes off without a glitch. I hope the kids enter into the worship. But these aren't the most important things to me. I choose to stand by the door and welcome each child by name, to give hugs, to speak words of encouragement. I choose to stand by the door as they leave, telling them I'm glad they came and that I'll be praying for them. It's the kids who count to me. I want them to know I love them and God loves them. This is a part of my career—my volunteer career—that allows me to make people a priority.

But what if you have a career that doesn't allow you to touch people directly? What if you sit at a computer, do your work in solitude, aren't in contact with the crowds? You can still touch people.

First, there are probably people who work with you and around you. Your coworkers, the mail carrier, the guy who brings bagels and coffee. Even if your career keeps you isolated in your basement, there's undoubtedly some time when you interact with others. It might be through phone calls, e-mail, letters, or occasional personal visits. Make these contacts count.

Second, there likely are many people who are positively affected by the product or service you provide. I've spent a number of years writing and editing curricula to be used by families or churches. I don't get to see the people who use what I've written, yet I know my work, my career, is making a difference.

Third, your family is one of your career priorities. They are the ones who suffer when you work too hard, when you put in longer hours than you should, when you put money and "success" ahead of people. If your career is that of being a parent, then it's easy to see how important your family is. But when you're chasing success in another field, families often get left behind. Make your family one of your highest priorities, not only in your career but in your life.

Consider your career and the people who are part of it. How are you making these people a priority? How can you make them more of a priority and let them know they're important to you?

WHAT'S IN YOUR JAR?

Let's go back to our science experiment. We have the jar of our career and we're putting in the stones that are top priorities. The stones that relate to the purpose of our career go into the jar. The stones that represent things we're passionate about go into the jar, along with those stones that represent tasks that must be done and in which we're going to choose to find delight. And then there's that big stone representing people, our biggest priority. After all these go in, the jar is pretty full! Now let's fill in the cracks with rice.

The smaller things in our careers are the ones that don't *have* to go in the jar. These are things that we could cut if we need more breathing room. The things that might bring stress and frustration if we overload on them. Things like taking on an extra project to make a good impression on a supervisor. Things like spending twenty-five hours making party decorations for a party where the kids are going to eat a cupcake and zoom to the swimming pool in five minutes (trust me, these things happen). Things like volunteering to do something because no one else has stepped forward. The "rice" activities are those we can choose to do *if we want to*.

I've noticed that a lot of us choose to do the jar experiment in reverse order. We fill up our careers with the rice—the things that don't really have to be done—then, as we try to cram the stones of priority into our lives, they don't fit.

Put in the priorities first, then fill in the cracks with the things of lesser importance.

Remember how I said I was going to leave water out of our experiment? Even though there were tiny spaces in between the grains of rice that still could be filled, these spaces don't *need* to be filled. In the same way, we don't need to fill every nook and cranny of our careers with things like negative opinions, carelessness, irritability, and so on. Leave these things out *completely!* And if other people try to force these unnecessary attitudes on you, confront them or keep away from them. Your career life is full and overflowing with abundance—there's no room for these fats!

Making choices requires us to weigh our options and select the best. Do this for your career. Trim away the excess fats of being overburdened, stressed, angry, and worn out. Then nurture the priorities of your career. You're on the right track! Let's keep moving!

NINE

The Low-Fat Checkbook

No one can serve two masters. Either he will hate the one
and love the other, or he will be devoted to the one and
despise the other. You cannot serve both God and Money.

—MATTHEW 6:24

Carla couldn't wait to show off her new fur coat.

"Feel how soft it is!" she exclaimed. "And it's really warm, too!"

I knew Carla and her husband were struggling financially as they, like Mike and me, worked their way through college. They wondered each month how they'd pay the electricity bill, so I was surprised by the fur coat and was blunt enough to ask, "How could you afford such a luxury?"

Carla's innocent response was, "We got a credit card in the mail! We had a $500 limit, and this coat cost only $450. We still have $50 to spend!"

Though I remained silent, I wanted to say, "I hate to break it to you, Carla, but that money was not a gift. You're going to have to pay it back— along with high interest."

It's easy to shake our heads ruefully at the naiveté of Carla and her husband. Yet most of us are guilty of having our own financial blind spots. As Americans, we are notorious for overspending, racking up huge debts, maxing out credit cards, and living beyond our means. In fact, if you have extra money left over at the end of the month, an emergency savings account, and a budget you actually live within, you are the rare exception in our society.

All this brings us to the low-fat checkbook, which might sound odd at first. After all, don't we *want* our wallets and bank accounts to be full and fat? Well, we do want them to be *full,* but not *fat.* Fat in the financial sense is debt, anxiety, being behind in our bills, working extra jobs and extra hours. It's a fat that adds tension to our homes and fear to our careers ("What if I lose my job?") and robs us of peace of mind. We've already worked to make the best choices in our homes and careers, so why should we now let financial fat weigh us down? Even as we've cleaned the fat of clutter out of our souls, financial stresses can add a new kind of fat and a sense of disarray to our lives.

Financial expert and best-selling author Suze Orman explains:

> In the purely financial realm, when our papers are cluttered and our affairs unattended to, we create a swirl of financial chaos around us. We bounce checks, we pay late charges on our mortgage, we forget to renew our driver's license or pay our property taxes. Why? We do this to obscure where we really stand, because we can't face our true financial selves, so we choose instead to ignore it, forget it, lose it, not face it—all actions that lead us away from money, not toward it, and keep us from creating.[1]

As a Christian, I want to be led toward God, not money. But it's even difficult to focus on a relationship with God when we've made choices that keep our thoughts on financial distress.

So how do we get that low-fat checkbook? How can we trim the fat of financial disorder and enjoy an abundance of what we need? Even though I'm not a financial guru, I've found guidance through books, articles, and the advice of others who are older and wiser than me. Add in a bit of personal experience, and I've found a number of truths that can help all of us master our money.

LIVE BELOW YOUR MEANS

In her book *The Courage to Be Rich,* Suze Orman tells about a time when she had considerable income and had gotten used to living an expensive lifestyle. Then, due to a devastating business situation, she found herself without income. Instead of changing her lifestyle, she kept on spending as if nothing had happened. It wasn't long before she was heavily in debt and very unhappy with her life. She finally realized, "I was living with the trappings of wealth, but had no money. I was living a lie."[2]

When we spend money we don't have, we are living a sort of lie. We're telling ourselves we can afford things that we really cannot. We're lying to ourselves.

People who spend more than they make each month are living *beyond* their means. Those who spend just what they make, no more or no less, live right *at* their means. To have a low-fat checkbook, we want to live *below* our means, spending less than we make each month and then using the difference wisely.

Living below our income level allows us to put money in savings and plan for emergencies such as job loss, medical expenses, or major car or household repairs. It allows us to give freely, above and beyond what God asks. It allows us to invest for our retirement years. It allows us to have less stress in our careers. In fact, some people choose to live so far below their means that they only need to work part-time to support themselves. Because of frugality and wise money management, they have an abundance of time to spend as they like.

Where are you living? Beyond, at, or below your means? You don't need to be a math expert to figure it out. If you, like the average American, are living beyond your means, the question is: How can you start living below your means? The answer: Create a budget, get and stay out of debt, give, and plan for your future.

CREATING A BUDGET

Get a sheet of notebook paper or a legal pad and a pen—it's time to create a budget. At the top of the paper, write your monthly after-tax income. Write it in bold figures so you can keep referring back to it. Under this, create twelve columns and label these for each month of the year. (The six-columns-per-page columnar pads found in office supply stores are ideal for this task.)

Down the left side of the paper, list all the things you spend money on every month: housing (rent or mortgage), groceries, transportation (car payment, fuel costs, fares for public transit), insurance, entertainment, savings accounts, clothing, education, tithe or charitable giving, utilities, and so on. Try to consider every cost you normally encounter, including pet costs, prescriptions, gifts, car maintenance and repairs, meals eaten out, and doctor visits.

Then get out a calculator, your checkbook, or a stack of bills that show what you typically spend in each of these areas, and start allotting your monthly income into the proper slots. Some of these will be easy, such as house payment or rent, car payment and average gas costs, and insurance. Other expenses, such as clothing and gifts, may vary from month to month. Estimate how much you think you're already spending and compare this to how much you can afford to spend if you keep expenditures below your monthly income. I doubt you'll be surprised at how quickly the money is spent!

As with other goals we address in the Low-Fat Lifestyle, achieving financial freedom is a matter of making wise choices and sticking to them. Looking at a budget helps us make choices about spending. A new car this year? Not in the budget. Gifts for Christmas? We did budget for that and need to stick with the amount we agreed to spend. A vacation? The budget allows for a long weekend at a nearby hotel, but not for a Caribbean cruise. A budget allows you to see everything in black and white and know precisely how money has been allocated for each catagory.

Another helpful idea that goes hand in hand with creating a household budget is recording your expenditures. This means writing down each expense to see if the amount you are actually spending is what you've allowed. For example, our family had a pretty standard grocery budget for several years. But a few months ago, we noticed we regularly needed to make exceptions to this amount. We began tracking how much we actually spent on groceries (counting the extra stops made during the week) and found it was much higher than we'd budgeted a couple of years back. It seems having a teenage boy directly correlates to higher grocery costs. We needed to adjust our budget based on actual spending.

Creating a budget and tracking your spending will help you make choices so you're able to live below your means. It's also one of the key strategies for controlling debt.

GETTING AND STAYING OUT OF DEBT

You've probably heard people refer to "good debt" and "bad debt." Good debt would be the mortgage on a house (provided it's within your means), capital to fund a new business, or a school loan. These are expenses that, at least in theory, will provide long-term gains, which justifies short-term debt plus interest. Owning a home can be a good investment. A business, if successful, can have a big payoff down the road. And education usually helps you advance in your career. All of these are expenses where, if necessary and within your means, debt may not be a fat.

Bad debt would be vacations paid for on credit, as well as clothing, meals at restaurants, gifts, and so on. These are things that we enjoy now but pay for later (and with considerable interest added). Most bad debt is put on credit cards, so let's start with them.

One study shows that the average American household has approximately ten credit cards and an average balance of seven thousand dollars on those credit cards.[3] If this is true for you, it would take you years to pay off these debts if you were to stop making any new purchases and made only the minimum monthly payment each month. What's worse, after adding in the amount paid in interest, you may end up paying two or three times the original amount of the initial purchase. That kind of financial bondage is the antithesis of the Low-Fat Lifestyle.

Make a plan to pay off your credit card debt. It may require that you meet with a debt or credit counselor. You may need to consolidate your credit card payments into one payment or focus on making higher payments on one card at a time until each card's balance has been cleared. That's the getting-out-of-debt part. The *staying*-out-of-debt part is this: Cut up all the cards but one. You read that correctly. Choose the one with the lowest interest rate or the one that's most widely accepted, and cut the others to shreds. Then hide that one card away. Don't carry it with you. Don't have it handy when you're out and about. Put it in a drawer and leave it there until you absolutely must use it.

Robert G. Allen, who has taught his financial techniques worldwide, explains,

> Statistics have shown that this simple exercise will automatically and almost effortlessly cut your living expenses by an average of 30 percent over the next twelve months. Why? Because credit cards provide easy access to purchasing power. If you remove the easy access, you remove the temptation to spend. Thus, your overall spending will automatically decline.[4]

Pay for your purchases with cash, and if you don't have enough cash, then don't make the purchase. It's that simple. A credit card that's not so easily accessible can be used for emergencies. By emergencies, I mean *emergencies:* when the car breaks down on vacation or when a relative passes away and you have to buy an expensive plane ticket. (Contrary to popular opinion, needing a new pair of white shoes for Easter Sunday is *not* an emergency.)

Staying out of debt means spending less. You may think there's no way you can cut the budget and spend less than you already do. Here are a few ways to cut expenses:

- Use coupons. Small savings add up.
- Have things repaired instead of replacing them.
- Buy in bulk the products you use regularly, such as toilet paper, cereal, laundry detergent.

- Put a "No Soliciting" sign on your door, and when phone sales-people call, politely ask them to remove your name from their lists. Better yet, have your phone number added to a "no-call" list.

- Plan ahead when you go shopping. Having a written list of what you need helps keep you from making impulse purchases.

- Skip the lattes and other designer coffee drinks. Make your own coffee at home and save four dollars a day.

- Drink water when eating out. If you're in the mood to splurge, ask for a slice of lemon.

- See movies and other shows at the afternoon matinees, which are usually half the cost of evening shows.

- Take your lunch to work. That six to ten dollars a day for eating out adds up fast (and food you make at home is likely to be low-fat).

- Save on gasoline costs (and driving time) by calling stores ahead of time to see if the items you're looking for are in stock.

- Look for a bank that doesn't include extra fees for checking, ATM, and so on.

- Avoid advertising for a while. Ads on television, magazines, and elsewhere only tempt you to spend—and add clutter to your home.

- Quit using cable television. Disconnect your cable or at least cut back on the premium channels. This will reduce costs while adding time for your family.

There are always ways to cut back on spending. If you're like me, you grew up with parents who constantly nagged you to turn off the lights, close the refrigerator door, and take shorter showers. I hated hearing those comments about saving money and natural resources as a child, but I say the same things to my own family today!

THE GIFT OF GIVING

The idea of faithful giving comes straight from God. Leviticus 27:30-33 explains that God's people were to give a tithe of everything they produced—their crops, their fruit, their money, their sheep. Also, tithing is mentioned many other times in the Bible. The dictionary tells us that a tithe is "a tenth part of something paid as a voluntary contribution."[5] Most Christians (including me) believe that the Bible instructs us to give one-tenth of our earnings to God.

There are those who argue and quibble over the concept of the tithe. Some feel the tithe was an Old Testament idea that doesn't apply anymore. Others think the tithe is really a manipulative tool that causes guilt. Some debate whether the 10 percent should be calculated before taxes or after taxes. It can get crazy with all these nitpicking opinions!

It's not my intent to persuade you to give a certain amount, but I do believe that a Low-Fat Lifestyle involves faithful, generous giving. Giving removes the fats of possessiveness and greed while filling our lives with healthy things like joy, satisfaction, mercy, and compassion.

Give Cheerfully

Some people might moan as they reach for their wallets, "Okay, fine. Enough already! I'll give." But if we give begrudgingly, we're certainly not demonstrating a heart of gratitude. My guess is that if we give to God as if we were giving up our teeth, then he probably doesn't want our gift. Imagine how you'd feel if someone gave you a birthday present while grimacing.

No joy for the giver *or* the receiver! As the apostle Paul reminds us, "Each man should give what he has decided in his heart to give, not reluctantly or under compulsion, for God loves a cheerful giver" (2 Corinthians 9:7). In other words, when it comes to giving, *attitude* is more important than *amount.*

The Bible gives us plenty of examples of people who gave—some with a proper attitude, some not. The first example is found in Genesis 4, where we read about Adam and Eve's first children, Cain and Abel. These young men brought their offerings to God, and for some reason God found favor with Abel's gift but not Cain's. We're not told exactly why God looked favorably on one and not the other, but my guess is that attitude was a key factor. I can't imagine that Cain was a cheerful guy to be around, because not long after this incident, he lured his brother out to a field and killed him. Hebrews 11:4 gives us another clue into the hearts of these men: "By faith Abel offered God a better sacrifice than Cain did. By faith he was commended as a righteous man, when God spoke well of his offerings." The issue was not the gifts Cain and Abel brought to God as much as the condition of their hearts and attitudes.

Another example, this time from the New Testament, is provided in Mark 12:41-44. Jesus was at the temple, sitting near the place where people contributed their offerings to God. He watched many rich people toss hefty sums of money into the treasury. Then he saw a poor widow. In my mind, I see her as a tiny old lady, but she could easily have been a young woman who had already lost her husband. Either way, she was obviously poor. She dropped only two coins into the treasury, coins worth less than a penny.

I'll be honest—if I were sitting near someone who dropped two coins into the offering plate, I'd probably think, *What a cheapskate* (unless that person was three years old). But Jesus could see into the heart and soul of this woman and said to his disciples, "I tell you the truth, this poor widow has put more into the treasury than all the others. They all gave out of their wealth; but she, out of her poverty, put in everything—all she had to live on" (verses 43-44).

This woman must have had great trust and faith in God to give all she had, no matter how small the gift looked in the eyes of others. And from Jesus' comments, it seems she was giving with joy and gratitude rather than from a begrudging attitude.

Give to Partner with God

A man at our church recently said that his wife "doesn't believe in tithing," so they don't give to the church. I'll admit my reaction to his comment was one of disbelief. I work with this couple's kids in our children's ministry, and though almost everyone who works in our ministry is an unpaid volunteer, there are still costs for curriculum, photocopying, craft materials, snacks, and heating or cooling the rooms. I thought, *Does this mother think all of this is free? Who does she think pays for all the things provided for her children?*

As the daughter of a former pastor, I know that even a pastor needs income to feed his family and pay the bills. When we give to our churches, we're supporting God's ministry. It's a way we can partner with God.

We also partner with God when we give to ministries beyond our local church and to missionaries who spread God's Word and love around the world. I love to think how exciting it must be for people in ministry to know those back at home are praying for them, contributing money to provide for their daily needs, and even sending gifts of encouragement to remind them how important their work is. Yet I hear what I consider horror stories from missionaries about the "gifts" they sometimes receive from us "generous" Christians back here in the land of comfort. One missionary told of being sent *used* tea bags.[6] Apparently, someone went to the trouble of drying out used tea bags and mailing them overseas. The giver must have thought, *Hey, life is bad there, so she won't mind having my leftovers.*

If we're giving thoughtfully and cheerfully, we won't be sending these kinds of gifts! But do consider how you can be a partner with God as you give. I have discovered great joy in giving anonymously to someone who I knew was hungry or cold, knowing that God was using me to touch this person's life. And I've been on the other end, when others have given our family money or groceries during times of great need.

Give to Be Blessed

As I said earlier, I've known great joy when I've given to others. Sometimes I think I get more out of giving than the person who receives the gift! This sounds like a selfish motive—give to be blessed—but it happens! God does bless us when we give. As Jesus said,

> Give, and it will be given to you. A good measure, pressed down,
> shaken together and running over, will be poured into your lap. For
> with the measure you use, it will be measured to you. (Luke 6:38)

We can't outgive God. When we give our time, our resources, and our finances, God gives back to us. I'm not saying if you give five dollars today, God will give you ten dollars tomorrow. What I'm saying is that God will somehow give you a greater blessing because of your willingness to give.

I've heard a few preachers take this principle out of context, trying to manipulate people into giving more to their ministry with promises of rewards to come. God never tries to manipulate us; he simply wants us to know the joy of giving, just as he wants someone else to know the joy of receiving.

PLANNING FOR THE FUTURE

The final thing we need to consider with regard to a low-fat checkbook is saving. When we live below our means, we're able to take the money that was left unspent and tuck it away. I like to look at savings in three categories: for short-term needs, for emergencies, and for long-term plans.

Short-Term Savings

Several years ago, one of our cars was falling apart. We had a choice: We could buy a car on credit by taking out a loan, or we could save for a car. Since we've made a commitment to keep away from the fat of debt, we opted to save up for the car. This meant that instead of making a car payment to a dealership or bank each month, we made that payment to ourselves. It also meant that instead of *paying* interest to a lender, we were *earning* interest while our money was in savings. In less than two years, we had the money we needed for the car we wanted. We had to wait, but we avoided going into debt.

In the same way, you and I can save money toward improvements on our homes, a special vacation, or a newer computer. If you borrow money for these, you're going to be making a payment each month anyway. Delay the purchase and make the payments to your short-term savings account instead. Then enjoy the abundance you've saved and spend without guilt or stress. That's the Low-Fat Lifestyle!

Emergency Savings

A number of years ago, Mike had to have emergency surgery. There were complications from the surgery, and Mike was unable to work for about six months. During this time he could barely get out of bed. I had been writing and editing only part time, mostly to bring in extra money for vacations or household items. Suddenly, the matter of our income was left to me.

We did have some savings, and because we didn't have any balance on our credit cards, we could use the savings if we needed to. (And, thankfully, we had friends with generous hearts.) God got us through this difficult time. I was grateful for the money we had in the bank and thankful that we didn't have debts to burden our lives. However, I wished then that we'd had *more* tucked away in savings for emergencies such as this.

With our roller-coaster economy, most of us live with concerns about being laid off, finding our income reduced due to cutbacks, or incurring large medical or repair bills. Whatever it is, it's a good idea to have several months' worth of income set aside as a cushion to fall back on. This is not money that you would use for a vacation or other optional purchase. It's set aside only for true needs. Some experts recommend having three months of income saved; others say six months is better. It may take a while to save up that much money, but work toward this goal. Hopefully, you'll never need this money. But if you do, you'll be thankful for your foresight!

Long-Term Savings

If you haven't started saving money for your retirement years, there's no time like the present. We can't count on the government to support us, so we need to make plans now for income in the later years of our lives. With

401(k)s, IRAs, Roth IRAs, SEP-IRAs, CDs, and a whole alphabet soup of other saving options, you're likely to find the best advice by meeting with a financial planner. This person can help you to select retirement savings plans—and appropriate investments to make within those plans—that enable you to save on a tax-advantaged basis and earn a fair amount of interest. Some of these accounts are also good for saving toward college for your children and other long-range goals.

I have family members who have planned well for their futures and can live without financial stress because they know they'll have a place to live and food on the table as they grow older. I also have family members who live with a high degree of stress and anxiety because they didn't plan ahead and are now suffering the consequences. Neither of these groups of people are better than the other or more or less deserving than the other— it's just that one planned ahead and the other did not. I hope you'll be one who plans ahead.

PART THREE

The Low-Fat Spirit

TEN

A Healthy Heart

And I pray that you, being rooted and established in love,
may have power, together with all the saints, to grasp how
wide and long and high and deep is the love of Christ, and
to know this love that surpasses knowledge—that you may
be filled to the measure of all the fullness of God.

—EPHESIANS 3:17-19

Imagine yourself involved in a world hunger relief effort. You've traveled
all the way to Africa and taken along loads of supplies. You're ready to feed
and serve the hungry. But when you arrive, the people appear to be robust
and healthy. What do you do?

This happened to author and speaker Jill Briscoe. She tells about a
time when she traveled to Africa, and the people her team had planned to
serve looked as healthy as could be.

Jill says, "When I got there I thought, *I've come to the wrong place.*
Everybody looked absolutely fine."

No one looked withered or malnourished. Had this been a colossal
mistake? Jill asked one of the leaders there what was going on.

"Jill, they're starving to death!" the man clearly assured her.

As Jill came to find out, the people farmed a kind of straw that looked similar to grain. They harvested it and made it into bread. But, she relates, "It had not one vitamin in it. It had not one food element in it. But it filled them up and actually built the fatty tissue.... It blew them up."[1]

Imagine it. People who look healthy but are actually starving to death. They're filling their stomachs with something that cannot nourish them. Eating this food staple staves off their hunger pangs even as it slowly leads to death.

For many people, this is exactly what happens in their spiritual life.

The spirit is the part of our being that's difficult for others to see. When it comes to our bodies, people can look at us and pretty much tell whether we've been eating low-fat foods. Likewise, people can look at the state of our homes and careers and tell if we're living a Low-Fat Lifestyle in these areas. Our physical appearance and many manifestations of our soul are open for others to view. But our spirit? That's another matter.

We can lie to others about our spiritual condition. We can even lie to ourselves. That's what the Pharisees of biblical times did. They put on a show of doing and saying all the right things. But Jesus called them "whitewashed tombs." Listen as he cries out to them:

> Woe to you, teachers of the law and Pharisees, you hypocrites! You are like whitewashed tombs, which look beautiful on the outside but on the inside are full of dead men's bones and everything unclean. In the same way, on the outside you appear to people as righteous but on the inside you are full of hypocrisy and wickedness. (Matthew 23:27-28)

Not exactly a compliment! These men had everyone else fooled. I can hear the people at the temple now: "Look at how holy those men are!

Why can't I be more like them? They've got it all together!" They had everyone fooled—even themselves! Yet Jesus looked into their hearts and saw their true spiritual condition. And it wasn't pretty. They were putting straw into their spirits and starving to death spiritually.

I certainly don't want to be the kind of person Jesus called a "whitewashed tomb." I don't want to look clean and happy on the outside while my spirit wastes away. I want to know God and know him fully. And I want my life to reflect that spiritual intimacy—not by piously *acting* good, but by actually *being* a godly woman. As with other areas of life, it comes down to the choices we make. Will we fill our spirit with fat or will we let it be nourished with God's fullness? More than any other choice we've talked about so far, I want the choices for my spirit to be the very best.

GOD'S GOODNESS IN FULL SUPPLY

In earlier chapters as we considered foods that are best to fill up on, we saw that fruits and vegetables—plants—were among our most healthful choices. Plants are created by God and are full of nutrition. Yet plants require only the basic goodness of God's creation to become filled with this nourishment. They need water, light, oxygen, and fertile soil—not much by our standards! And God provides all of these for them.

This theme is woven throughout the Scriptures. In Luke 12, we read Jesus' words,

Consider how the lilies grow. They do not labor or spin. Yet I tell you, not even Solomon in all his splendor was dressed like one of these. If that is how God clothes the grass of the field, which is here today, and tomorrow is thrown into the fire, how much more will he clothe you, O you of little faith! (verses 27-28)

If God takes care of the basic needs of the plants, how much more will he care for us?

Plants offer us a helpful metaphor as we consider how to apply the principles of the Low-Fat Lifestyle to our spirit. They require little, and what they do need is provided by God. And what they fill up on produces wholesome nutrition for others.

THE LESSON OF THE SEED

Jesus used many references to farming and plants to illustrate his spiritual lessons. Let's examine one of his parables, recorded in three different gospels (Matthew 13, Mark 4, and Luke 8). The story features a farmer who goes into his fields one morning and starts tossing handfuls of seed here and there. His method was to fling the seeds, let them fall where they may, and wait to see which ones would germinate and grow into healthy plants.

As Jesus tells it, some of the seed didn't last long on the soil because birds came and ate them. Also, people walked in the field and trampled some of the seed (apparently they hadn't heard of scarecrows and little signs saying "Keep off the grass"). This seed didn't have a chance.

More of the seed fell onto rocky places that didn't have much soil. With a little rain, this seed sprouted. Then the sun shined. But because these plants had no roots to carry moisture to the leaves, they became scorched and withered and then died.

Some other seed fell into soil that allowed it to sprout and grow. But along with the plants came weeds, which used up much of the water necessary for growth. Soon, the seedlings were crowded out and more of the farmer's plants shriveled and died.

But there was also seed that fell on good soil. This seed was able to enjoy the thirst-quenching water and bask in the warming sun. It grew strong. In fact, it grew so strong that it produced fruit—more fruit than anyone could have imagined, as well as more seed that could be planted for another harvest.

Jesus concluded this story with the comment, "He who has ears, let him hear" (Matthew 13:9).

No doubt some of Jesus' listeners walked away scratching their heads, wondering why Jesus was so interested in the fate of seeds. Others might have been cleaning out their ears, thinking, *Maybe I missed something. What was the point of that anecdote?* And there may have been a few for whom the meaning of the story was clear. It seems that the disciples were a bit confused, so Jesus explained what it all meant, and naturally, there's an application for us, too.

The Stolen Seed

The seed in this story, Jesus explained, refers to God's Word, the message of the gospel. When this message of love is spread about, it falls in many places. It's heard, felt, and observed by many, with varying results.

Just as some of the seed was quickly devoured by birds or trampled underfoot, some people hear the message of God's love and, because their hearts are so hard, the impact is lost. It doesn't take root. The Bible tells of those who have hardened their hearts against God, such as the Egyptian pharaoh, who refused to let the Israelites go, and the Pharisees, who could clearly see the love and mercy of Jesus yet refused to believe in him.

Have you ever seen this happen? Perhaps you've shown kindness to someone as a way of expressing God's love, and this person responded coldly or rudely. Or maybe you've shared how Jesus came to save us from the penalty we deserve, and a cynical person has made mocking comments. Each of us can probably think of several situations in our lives where someone has demonstrated a hard heart, a heart that isn't open to receiving the gifts God wants to lavishly give.

In his book *The Voice of the Heart,* Chip Dodd addresses how our hearts become hardened toward God:

> By rejecting our hearts and denying their contents, we have
> become spindly bushes living in resignation, steeped in denial,
> rationalization, and manipulation.… To hide our hearts, we work
> to acquire defenses so that our hearts can't be touched. We lower
> our spiritual and emotional expectations. We don't expect much
> from ourselves. We pretend we don't need much from others. And
> we deny how much we distrust and need God.[2]

I hope this doesn't describe you, hiding your heart from God with a variety of defenses. I hope you haven't let the frustrations and cruelty of the world harden you to God's love and care for you. If you do find yourself becoming callous and closing your ears to God as he calls you to himself, I encourage you to pray humbly for a renewed spirit. Ask God to tenderly knead your hardened spirit and make it pliable again. Let us never turn our hearts away from the greatest love we'll ever know!

The Rootless Seed

Jesus went on to explain that the seed that fell upon rocky soil represents those who hear the message and receive it with joy. But without roots, the message is soon lost for these people. As Jesus put it, "When trouble or persecution comes because of the word, he quickly falls away" (Matthew 13:21).

This makes me think of people who, in a wave of emotion, commit their lives to Jesus. For a few days, they're filled with excitement and joy. Then they realize their friends haven't made the same decision. They find that others aren't welcoming them with open arms anymore. They might hear, "You've changed—we want the old you back." And these people buckle under the pressure. Without having their faith nurtured, without time spent soaking up God's Word, these changed hearts shrivel up and return to their old ways.

I can think of several celebrities who have claimed to be changed by Christ and then disclaimed him a short time later. These people are put under great scrutiny by the media, by society, even by cynical Christians. No one takes them in and says, "Let me help you grow." Just as the heat of the sun bombarded the seedlings in Jesus' story, the heat of the spotlight scorches these people. And without the life-giving moisture of love and God's Word, they have nothing from which to draw strength. They wilt and turn away from the joy they had found.

Of course, this happens to many people who aren't celebrities. Maybe it's happened to you. You've wanted to believe. You've wanted to grow. But you haven't learned how to put down roots. Or perhaps no one has come alongside to nurture you, to help you come to know God as a friend. If this is true for you, now is the time to put down roots. Now is the time to soak up the words of the Bible. Now is the time to bask in prayer and worship. If you don't know how, keep reading because we're going to address these important privileges in the coming chapters. Don't turn away. Don't become frustrated. Don't let the rocks in your life keep you from drinking deeply from the well of God's love.

The Fat-Choked Seed

Jesus explained what he meant by the plants that grew among thorns that choked them and kept them from bearing fruit. These were hearts that heard the message, were well watered, and began to grow. But then...

> the worries of this life and the deceitfulness of wealth choke it,
> making it unfruitful. (Matthew 13:22)

> the desires for other things come in and choke the word.
> (Mark 4:19)

> as they go on their way they are choked by life's worries, riches
> and pleasures, and they do not mature. (Luke 8:14)

As Jesus puts it, the "fats" of life choke this growing faith and keep it from maturing. Worry, the pursuit of wealth, desires for other things, the pursuit of pleasures—all of these keep our spirit from growing. Remember Jesus' words: He said he came to give us life in all its fullness (see John 10:10). He doesn't want us to have a halfhearted faith, a wimpy heart, an immature spirit. God wants us to grow to fullness, to maturity, to the point where we can bear fruit.

It's my guess that most of us can see ourselves in this description at least some of the time. We love God and want to grow, but other things compete for our affections. We have worries, we're busy, we're distracted. Our minds are on our careers or our finances. We've got dinner in the oven, there's a new sitcom on television, the kids are calling, and the boss is putting on the pressure. Who's got time for God in the midst of all that? So, despite good intentions, we allow the thorns and weeds of life to choke out our greatest love.

"As a matter of fact, I *am* busy," you might be saying. "But I'm busy with important things—things I wouldn't call 'thorns.' I'm serving on the PTA, teaching Sunday school, earning a living, taking time to exercise—all things that are priorities. Why the guilt trip?"

Remember what we've been saying. A healthy, wholesome, Low-Fat Lifestyle is achieved by making wise choices. Even in the midst of all the good things, even in the midst of the best things, we must choose to spend time with God. We must choose to grow in spiritual maturity instead of letting the other priorities of life choke out the abundant life he has in store for us.

The Healthy Seed

Finally, we come to the seed that fell on good soil. Jesus said this seed represented the hearts that heard the word, understood it, accepted it, and then produced a bountiful crop. In his own words, "But the seed on good soil stands for those with a noble and good heart, who hear the word, retain it, and by persevering produce a crop" (Luke 8:15).

Wouldn't you love it if Jesus described you as someone with a noble and good heart? What if he said you are someone who is producing a spiritual crop greater than what was originally sown in your heart? Wouldn't it be awesome to hear Jesus say that you kept the message in your heart through good times and bad and now you're helping others mature in the faith?

Let's choose to avoid the "fats" of hard hearts, rocky soil, thorns, and weeds. Let's make sure we're firmly rooted in fertile soil that enables us to mature and produce a bountiful crop.

Developing a low-fat spirit is the most exciting part of our journey together, because it's the part that matters most. Though low-fat eating is important, our bodies will pass away. Though streamlining our family life, finances, and careers will help us live more fully, our earthly pursuits will fade away. But our spirit is eternal. Though friends and neighbors can't see what's going on inside us, God certainly can. He calls us first and foremost to nurture this aspect of our lives—to trim away anything that would impede our spiritual growth while we fill up on worship, prayer, his Word, and involvement with the family of God.

ELEVEN

Filling Up on Worship and Prayer

Come near to God and he will come near to you.

—JAMES 4:8

A few years ago, my son, Tony, and I took a trip with my parents while Mike remained at home due to work. It was during the middle of the summer, and things get dry and hot in Colorado, so I left a detailed watering schedule for Mike: "On Monday, water the front yard and flower beds on the side of the house. On Tuesday, water the backyard and the flowers in the border area…"

When we returned ten days later, I was dismayed to find the grass brown and my flowers dead. Not just wilted—they were all crumble-in-your-fingers dry. I was deeply disappointed. Sure, they were just flowers, but I'd put so much time and effort into nurturing them. Mike weakly explained that it had rained while we were gone, and he thought that would be enough for the plants. Later, the neighbors told me it had sprinkled for several minutes one afternoon, and that was about it. Besides, even a long rain wouldn't have helped all the *indoor* plants that were also dead.

Water. H_2O. Without it, every living thing will die. Water makes up between 50 to 90 percent of living organisms and is, in essence, the lifeblood for much of what God created. It provides nourishment. It quenches our thirst. It washes us, refreshes us, relaxes us.

In Jesus' parable that we examined in the last chapter, it was essential for the seed to fall on good soil—the fertile soil of our hearts. But no matter how willing and open our hearts are, if we don't provide the right sustenance, the seed will wither and die. In our spiritual lives, the "water" that promotes growth and development includes studying God's Word and fellowshiping with other believers (which we'll discuss in subsequent chapters). And there are two more essential elements: prayer and worship. Without these two sources of nourishment, our spirit can become parched; with them, we can thrive and flourish.

THE ESSENCE OF PRAYER AND WORSHIP

Before we go further, let's take a moment to consider what prayer and worship are. In the simplest of terms, prayer is talking or communicating with God. Through prayer, we can thank God for the great works he has done both in our lives and in the lives of others. Through prayer, we can pour out our hearts to our heavenly Father, sharing our deepest fears, needs, and concerns. We can admit the wrongs we've done and commit to repent—turn away from—our sins. There's nothing we can't share with God through prayer.

God already knows what's on our hearts, but he longs for us to share everything with him. When my son comes home from school, I could look through his papers to find out about his day, but I'd rather hear all the details from his own lips. Our relationship grows stronger through this kind of interaction. God wants that kind of two-way relationship with us, and it's built through communication.

Worship is a kind of prayer, but the focus is not on our needs and desires. When we worship, we communicate to God how awesome and wonderful he is. We show honor and reverence. Worship takes our minds off ourselves and turns our hearts to God. It is simply praising God because he is God. And while worship is for God, we benefit from it as well. As Thomas Aquinas said, "We pay God honor and reverence, not for his sake (because he is of himself full of glory to which no creature can add anything), but for our own sake."[1]

Some people think it's a bit odd that God wants us to tell him how great he is. Doesn't he already know? Is he so insecure that he needs us to constantly affirm him? Not at all! Worship is our response to the greatness of God.

When I'm on a car trip with my mother, she can't help but constantly comment on the beauty of nature as we drive. "Look at the snow-covered mountains!" she gasps. "And do you see those tiny yellow flowers out there in the desert? Gorgeous! Simply gorgeous!"

Our family teases her about this, but it's a good example of how we should respond to God. Mom can't keep quiet about the beauty she sees—it's a natural response for her. Likewise, worship is our natural response to the beauty of God. Popular worship leader Matt Redman puts it this way: "The heart of God loves a persevering worshipper who, though overwhelmed by many troubles, is overwhelmed even more by the beauty of God."[2] No matter what life looks like around us, we can turn our eyes to God and be moved to worship him.

Think of a young husband telling his new wife how beautiful she is. She's filled with joy at his words and his recognition of something about her that others may not see. The man experiences the joy of knowing he's lifted her up, the joy of knowing her heart is made glad. And the bond between them is strengthened. Worship does that for us. We give joy to God through worship, we experience the overflow of that joy in our own lives, and our intimacy with God grows.

So how are prayer and worship like water for our spiritual lives? Read on, and let's find out!

OUR NEED FOR NOURISHMENT

I heard about a little boy who misbehaved and was sent to bed immediately. After being in his room for a few minutes, the boy called out to his father, "Dad, will you bring me a drink of water?"

"No," replied the father. "You're being punished. Now go to sleep."

A few minutes later, the boy hollered again. "Dad, I'm really thirsty. Please bring me a drink of water."

"Listen, young man," the father said, "if I hear one more peep out of you, I'm coming in there to spank you. Go to sleep!"

Silence lasted only a couple of minutes. Then the boy called again, "Dad, when you come in here to spank me, will you bring me a drink of water?"

Like that boy, we have all had times when we were *really* thirsty. When we feel parched, our bodies tell us that we've *got* to have something to drink. And of course, it's not just when we feel thirsty that we need water; we need it continually. There's a constant need. I believe the same is true of prayer and worship—our spirit has a constant need for them. Indeed, we were created to worship.

Imagine a rock concert or a huge sporting event. The fans respond to the musicians or athletes with cheers, raised hands, even tears of emotion. Fans dress in clothing that associates them with their idols, and they buy coffee mugs, jewelry, backpacks, bumper stickers, and other items that bear the images or logos of these stars. Fans also learn the most intricate details of the stars' personal lives, or they memorize obscure facts and statistics about teams and their performances.

Millions of people in our culture worship celebrities and pop icons. Just as it's natural for us to get thirsty, it seems as if we have an inborn desire to worship. But when we don't worship God, we find something else to fill the void. Unfortunately, the substitutes are temporary and are not truly deserving of our worship. They don't quench our spiritual thirst. So we remain hollow, unfilled, and spiritually thirsty.

I'm sure everyone has heard that it's best for our bodies to have at least eight glasses of water a day. That's a lot of water! Some people try to fill this need by drinking coffee, sodas, milk, or juice, but nutritionists tell us that these substitutes do not provide the nourishment and cleansing effect of plain water.

Or think of your garden. You wouldn't water your tomato plants with Pepsi or lemonade. In order for the plants to flourish, you water them with…*water*.

The first of the Ten Commandments tells us we're not to worship any other god but the one true God. This command is repeated throughout the Bible. Our bodies have a constant need for pure water, and our spirits have a constant need for the pure and true God. The Scriptures remind us of the constancy of this need:

I will extol the LORD at all times; his praise will always be on my lips. (Psalm 34:1)

Be joyful always; pray continually; give thanks in all circumstances, for this is God's will for you in Christ Jesus. (1 Thessalonians 5:16-18)

To help us grow closer to God each day and thrive in his love, peace, and joy, God instructs us to constantly drink the water of prayer and worship. Are you giving your spirit the nourishment it needs? Are you spending time each day talking with God? Are you worshiping him as a way of life?

Refreshment for a Parched Spirit

Do you remember those old iced-tea commercials where someone would take a drink and then fall backward into a pool of water? How refreshing! When our mouths are dry and parched, nothing sounds better than being drenched with water.

Now imagine being spiritually dry. Think of those times when you felt as if your prayers were hitting the ceiling of your bedroom and sticking there. Think of the times that you felt pushed down or rejected, alone or desperate. Those are the times when you need the refreshment that only prayer and worship can bring.

One recent Sunday I felt drained due to a family illness. I felt empty and hopeless. I didn't want to go to church that day, but I had responsibilities, so I went, thinking I'd leave as soon as my part was done. Everyone was singing as I entered the sanctuary, and to be honest, I groaned inwardly. I had nothing to sing about that day. Yet just listening to the words of the song and hearing others praise God made my heart feel lighter. The song spoke of God's presence raining down on us and healing us. I began to sing the words, trying to mean what I sang. I longed for the words to be true. And they became true. As I turned my focus away from my own problems and toward God's power, my heart was refreshed. My attitude was changed. In giving to God, he gave back to me.

Others have shared similar experiences with me. They've felt as if God was far away and they were stagnant and spiritually dry. Yet when they began to worship God, their hearts and attitudes were changed. They were refreshed by giving praise.

The Bible tells us that prayers of repentance also bring refreshment to our spirit. Acts 3:19 says, "Repent, then, and turn to God, so that your sins may be wiped out, that times of refreshing may come from the Lord."

In what ways do you need to be refreshed? A Low-Fat Lifestyle is one in which we regularly shed the burden of sin through repentance and receive God's nourishment. Ask God for this refreshment, and experience the abundance only he can provide.

A Means of Transport

We've talked about water as an element that brings about growth and provides refreshment. Here's another wonderful thing about water: It is a means of transport. Ships carry cargo across lakes or oceans. Supplies are sent by boats down rivers. Even within our bodies, water is the basis of our blood that transports what is needed through our system and removes impurities. Through the flow of water we are kept healthy.

Similarly, we are kept spiritually healthy through the flow of worship and prayer. These practices transport us, or move us, into a deeper relationship with God. By listening to him and sharing with him, we move closer to him.

Another way we're kept healthy is through the removal of waste. Without getting too graphic, let's just say that water removes waste from living beings, whether plant or animal. It softens blockages and transports what's no longer needed (or was never needed). Through prayer and worship we allow God to remove the waste from our spirits. When we ask God to eliminate the sin and wastes in our hearts, he does. Talk to God about this, allow him to transport that waste away from your heart, then praise him for his incredible ability to do so.

A Cleanser for the Spirit

During many of my growing-up years, my family lived near the beach. When we'd get home from our hours of jumping in the water, digging for crabs, and building sandcastles, my parents wouldn't let us in the house until we'd gone into the backyard and hosed off. The sand was everywhere, clinging to our sweaty, salty bodies. But just a moment under the spray of the garden hose would rinse the sand away.

Prayer is like a hose that cleans us. The psalmist asked God to "wash away all my iniquity and cleanse me from my sin" (51:2). It is not our prayers that purify us but rather the God to whom we pray. It is he who washes us and makes us pure.

There's also the *feeling* of being cleansed that comes through prayer and worship. When we've sinned and know we need forgiveness, there's a feeling of cleansing that comes when we ask God to wash our hearts. There's also the clean feeling that comes through worship, through being in the presence of a holy God. People have told me they didn't feel like they should be worshiping because they were feeling guilty over their actions of the week. That's a time when we *need* to worship and pray, to let God's Spirit cleanse us.

A Solvent for Hardened Hearts

I'm sure this has happened to you many times: You're washing the dishes and come to a crusty spot of burned sauce in a pan. You can scrub and scour for half an hour, or you can let it soak. I usually go for the soaking option, since it's a lot easier! Water is the universal solvent. It softens and dissolves all kinds of hardened elements.

Prayer and worship can work like solvents in our hearts. Through prayer, God can soften our hearts so we can hear his words. Our own worries can be dissolved and carried away, to be cared for by God. I like how Charles Swindoll puts it:

> What comes from the Lord because it is impossible for humans to manufacture it? Wisdom. What comes from humans because it is impossible for the Lord to experience it? Worry. And what is it that brings wisdom and dispels worry? Worship.[3]

Worry and doubt are fats we don't need. Yet these are things that are tougher to eliminate than, say, a tablespoon of butter. They have to be dissolved or removed for us. When we fill our spirit with prayer and worship, the fats that we can't control are dissipated. God fills us instead with comfort, peace, wisdom, joy, and other good things.

WORSHIP: DIFFERENT FORMS, DIFFERENT STYLES

Every schoolchild learns that water has three forms: liquid, solid, and gas. Water, ice, and steam. Water doesn't always look the same. Neither do prayer and worship.

Some people pray aloud, others in silence. Prayers can be as artistic as poetry or as unadorned as a cry for help. We can worship alone, with a few others, or in the company of thousands. There is no one formula for prayer and worship, and variety adds to our spiritual experience.

Jesus prayed alone and he prayed with the masses. Some people in the Bible bowed or fell on their faces before God as they prayed or worshiped. David danced as he praised God. The Psalms are full of references to singing praises to God, as well as using instruments to worship noisily or beautifully. Other times, we're encouraged to be still and meditate on God's beauty. The Bible doesn't say we should always bow our head and fold our hands or sing only the songs in our hymnals. God created us to be like him—creative!

One form of worship that's often overlooked is *serving* God. Romans 12:1 says, "Therefore, I urge you, brothers, in view of God's mercy, to offer your bodies as living sacrifices, holy and pleasing to God—this is your spiritual act of worship." Since God has been merciful and kind to us, we can and should demonstrate these same qualities toward others. Offering our bodies to serve God with our talents, resources, and time is a form of worship.

Are you looking for a little variety in your prayer and worship life? Here are a few ideas:

- Go for a walk alone. Talk to God and listen for him in the silence.
- Shout your praise to God. (You may have to go into the garage or sit in your car to find a place where people won't stare.)
- Put on your favorite worship album, turn up the stereo, and sing praises to God at the top of your voice.
- Write your prayers in a journal. Reflect on how God has worked in the past as you read over previous entries. Thank God for the answers to prayer you've seen.
- Write a poem of worship.
- Read the Psalms and reflect on the prayers and praises offered there.

- Be still. Fill your mind with thoughts of God's greatness and power.

- Kneel as you talk to God. This demonstrates humility and allegiance to the King.

- Listen to children laughing and join in. Consider Psalm 100:1: "Make a joyful noise unto the LORD, all ye lands" (KJV). And think on Psalm 89:15: "How blessed are the people who know the joyful sound!" (NASB). What sound is more joyful than laughter?

- And remember that God loves a cheerful giver (2 Corinthians 9:7). We usually think of this in terms of giving financially. But God also wants us to offer our prayers and praises with cheerful hearts.

FEEL THE POWER

There's no doubt that water has incredible power. Think of the crashing waves of the ocean and how they can reduce a ship to splinters. Or imagine the devastating power of rushing water that can tear through a town and wipe away buildings, cars, or anything else in its path. The power of water has been harnessed to generate electricity. Even a trickle of water has the ability to, over time, smooth the roughest stone.

Similarly, prayer and worship have incredible power. I cannot list the times my own life has been changed by the power of prayer. God has done things I never would have thought possible through the prayers of those I know. And I can't even begin to imagine all that God has done through the prayers of Christians over hundreds of years and throughout the world. It's an overwhelming thought!

In Acts 16, we see a great example of the power of worship and prayer. Here we read how Paul and Silas commanded a demon to leave a young girl who had been used by her owners as a fortune-teller. Fearing a loss of their income, the owners were furious. They grabbed Paul and Silas and literally dragged them to the authorities to make their complaint. The two were stripped, cruelly beaten, shackled, and put into jail with extra guards.

Under those circumstances, you might have expected Paul and Silas to defend their actions or complain about the injustice of it all. You might even have expected them to grumble at how God had let them down. But no, they praised him. Verse 25 says they were "praying and singing hymns to God, and the other prisoners were listening to them." Paul and Silas's prison mates might have thought they were crazy—or found them inspirational. We don't know. We do know that in the middle of the night, God caused an earthquake. The prisoners were freed! Instead of running away, however, Paul and Silas stayed and led the jailer and his entire household to Christ.

God works when we pray. God works when we worship. Where do you need to see God's power? Pray about it. And then worship, even if the situation you're praying about doesn't change. God can change your situation, or he can change your attitude and perspective. He's that powerful.

Our hearts need to be washed, refreshed, awakened, and changed by prayer and worship. When we fail to consistently engage in these life-changing disciplines, we allow fats such as discontent, hopelessness, and indifference into our lives. Just as a plant cannot live without the nourishment of water, our spirit cannot live without the pure water of prayer and worship.

TWELVE

Filling Up on God's Word

Your word is a lamp to my feet and a light for my path.

—PSALM 119:105

God, come out of the hole!"

The native warrior leaned over a deep hole he had dug, shouting with excruciating, agonizing cries. Over and over he yelled, "God, God, come out of the hole!"

Deep in the jungles of South America, a puzzled missionary named Bruce Olson carefully approached this man whom he knew to be both brutal and adept with a bow and arrow. Bruce dared to ask the man why he was calling to God in the hole. Others explained that the man's brother had died from the bite of a poisonous snake, and since the brother had died away from his home, it was believed that his spirit would never go to "God beyond the horizon."

The man was looking for God in order to plead with him, to see if God would give the brother breath again so his spirit would not be lost. The man didn't know where to find God, and he figured a hole was as good a place to look as any other. He was desperate and hopeless.

As Bruce talked to the men gathered there, natives of a tribe called the

Motilones, one man mentioned a legend of their people that told of a "prophet who would come carrying banana stalks, and that God would come out of those stalks." Bruce pondered this statement, and in the silence another man walked over to a banana stalk and cut it. The leaves folded out like pages, and Bruce realized the "banana stalk" was the Bible. God truly could "come out" of the pages of the Bible and meet these people. Bruce held out his Bible and said, "This is it! I have it here! This is God's banana stalk."

One of the men grabbed the Bible from Bruce and began tearing out the pages and stuffing them into his mouth! He wanted to have God inside him and figured eating the "banana stalk" would be the surest way to achieve this. Bruce stopped the man and explained that God's Word could be taken in by *hearing,* not eating, the message. Through careful conversation, Bruce used the practices and lore of the Motilones to share the love of God with these people who longed to know him. They finally were able to know God through the banana stalk—the Bible.[1]

Thankfully, we don't have to eat the Bible, but we do need to fill up on it regularly. We need to hear it, read it, study it. That's how we get to know God.

We know that plants need fertile soil and plenty of water to grow, just as our hearts need to be fertile to God's message and strengthened through prayer and worship. What else do plants need? Light. Heat. Energy. In our physical world, these crucial elements are provided by the sun. So as we continue with our metaphor using plants to illustrate our spiritual needs, we'll use the sun to represent the need for God's Word, the Bible, in our lives.

LET THERE BE LIGHT

Think back to your grade-school days and those science fairs that were held each year. There was always one kid (maybe it was you) who did a project with lights and plants. This budding biologist would put one plant in the sun, one in the dark, and maybe a few others in places that received various amounts of light. The final project would show a few withered plants along with a healthy one. The simple lesson? Plants need a daily dose of light.

Now if this same biology whiz did a report with his or her experiment, it would mention photosynthesis. This is the process, you'll recall, in which plants use light to change carbon dioxide and water into glucose. Glucose then provides energy for the plant to grow, and as a by-product of photosynthesis, oxygen is created. (Isn't God's creation amazing?) According to one encyclopedia, "Virtually all life on earth, directly or indirectly, depends on photosynthesis as a source of food, energy, and oxygen, making it one of the most important biochemical processes known."[2]

Without the sun, without light, there would be no life and no growth.

Light has many other important purposes as well. We need light to help us see where we're going and where we've been. Light shows us where the bumps and potholes are in the road ahead. And as light reflects off our faces, we are said to "glow" and "shine."

The Bible is a lot like light in all of these ways.

A Source of Guidance

Have you ever been camping and had to walk along a twisty dirt path to the bathroom at night? (This is why I never go camping.) On a dark night, you need a flashlight to get you where you're going. Or what about the times at home when the power goes out and the house is plunged into darkness? You need a candle so you don't trip and fall. Our spiritual lives are like that. We need the light of God's Word to guide us through the dark times—and even the not-so-dark times. The Bible itself teaches us that the words of God guide us:

Direct me in the path of your commands, for there I find delight. (Psalm 119:35)

Your word is a lamp to my feet and a light for my path. (Psalm 119:105)

For these commands are a lamp, this teaching is a light. (Proverbs 6:23)

When we're unsure what direction we should go in life, the Bible is our guide. Now it's true that the Bible doesn't say, "You should quit your job and train to become a dentist," or "The blue blouse matches the skirt you're going to wear today." These are choices that are left up to us (even if we are in the dark as to what's fashionable these days). Instead, the Bible guides us by telling us what God is like, how to treat others, what is moral and what is immoral, and so on. The Ten Commandments are guides for how to live, and the Gospels guide us to salvation. The Bible offers information and insights so we can develop purity, joy, courage, peace, maturity…well, the list could go on for pages.

Most likely you've reached decision points in your life when you didn't know what to do. Some people randomly flip open the Bible, put their finger on a verse, and take the message as God's instruction to them. You have to be careful when using that method. After all, you might find yourself moving to Egypt or something equally unhelpful.

A better approach is to consider passages that help you determine if one path is right and another is wrong. Or if one will take you away from something important, such as your family or even God. Even if you can't find a passage that gives you clear direction, you're certain to find words of peace and encouragement. Turn to the Bible for light when things seem dark around you, and enjoy it even when life is filled with light.

Words of Warning

That same flashlight you relied on to guide you to the campground bathroom might also shine upon the beady eyes of a skunk. Warning! Go the other way! And the intense glare of a lighthouse beacon makes it clear that danger is ahead for ships that continue toward the rocks. Even the faintest nightlight will keep you from stepping on your child's LEGOs when you go in to give the little angel a good-night kiss. Light lets us see things ahead that we want to avoid. It warns us where we shouldn't step. The Bible does this for us too.

For example, the book of Proverbs warns us of the dangers of gossip, laziness, dishonesty, pride, a quick temper, and more. When we see these things in our lives or in the lives of those we spend time with, we know there will be danger ahead unless we change course.

Galatians 5:19-21 is another place where the Bible guides us away from danger:

The acts of the sinful nature are obvious: sexual immorality, impurity and debauchery; idolatry and witchcraft; hatred, discord, jealousy,

fits of rage, selfish ambition, dissensions, factions and envy; drunken-
ness, orgies, and the like. I warn you, as I did before, that those who
live like this will not inherit the kingdom of God.

If these qualities or activities are in our lives, then we need to clear them
out or suffer the consequences.

Many places in the Bible tell us what things to avoid and keep out of
our lives. Not that the Bible is a list of don'ts. It simply lets us know that
if we fill our lives with wrong actions and attitudes, then we're heading
into a trap.

A Bright Reflection

My son has a number of plastic glow-in-the-dark stars stuck to his bedroom ceiling. During the day these stars soak up the light from his windows. At night that stored light faintly shines. This happens to us when
we fill up on the Bible. We soak it up as we read. We shine with the light
that's inside us, and it is reflected in our lives. Consider these passages:

The light of the righteous shines brightly, but the lamp of the
wicked is snuffed out. (Proverbs 13:9)

You are the light of the world. A city on a hill cannot be hidden.
Neither do people light a lamp and put it under a bowl. Instead
they put it on its stand, and it gives light to everyone in the
house. In the same way, let your light shine before men, that they
may see your good deeds and praise your Father in heaven.
(Matthew 5:14-16)

When we fill our hearts with God's Word, we can't help but shine! And when we radiate with the Lord's love and joy, we'll lead others to him. Tony's glowing stars are pale imitations of the sun, but they do give back a tiny bit of the light. We pale in comparison to God, but when we soak up his Word, we can reflect some of that light to guide others.

When I was in high school, a teacher once said to me, "There's something different about you. What is it?" At the time I was so flustered that I stammered something about being cheerful most of the time, but I knew right away what this man was getting at. God's love was shining through me. I wish I'd been ready to share that message instead of giving a lame answer. So learn from my blunder and be ready to share as you shine.

Joy Comes in the Morning

I have never been to a hospital emergency room during the day. The doctors and nurses I've seen there at night have never seen me wearing anything other than sweats; they've never seen me with my hair combed, and they've often seen me with baby vomit and other gross substances smeared on my clothes. Why do we always seem to be the sickest at night? And why is it always so scary to be sick at night? Most parents can recall nights they've spent awake with sick children, thinking through those hours, *Will the night ever end?* During those miserable, lonely, and frightening hours, we long for the light of day when all will seem well again.

I don't imagine Daniel was given a light when he was tossed into the lions' den. After all, he was on his way to certain death. At the time, Daniel had no way of knowing what the morning light would hold for him—he was just hoping to see it. It must have been a long, dark night.

The Bible has a verse for nights like those: "Weeping may endure for a night, but joy comes in the morning" (Psalm 30:5, NKJV). With the light of day, our tears cease and we feel peace and joy again. The light of the Bible brings us joy, especially after times of pain and turmoil.

Mike and I lost two babies before they were born. The days and months after those sad events were filled with weeping. And even though I never could find an answer for my sadness, I did find peace and comfort through God's Word. Eventually, I even found joy again. I would not have found joy on my own or by filling up on feel-good books and magazine articles. I needed to daily fill my spirit with God's messages to me. And while I hope you don't have times of great sadness in your life, I'm realistic enough to know there will be times when you're longing for the light of day to break through so you can find that joy again too. Find it by filling up on God's Word. It's truly the only message that will heal your heart.

TURN UP THE HEAT

There's something so pleasant about sitting in the warm sunshine. Even our dog, a tiny Chihuahua, somehow manages to find the one spot on the floor where the sun is shining through the window. That's where she curls up and goes to sleep. I need more than a tiny spot of sun, so I pull open the curtains to let in the warm sunlight.

In Colorado the winters are cold, so when spring and summer arrive, it's so relaxing to sit in a sunny spot and feel the warmth of the sun's rays. That heat is comforting, warming. And when heat gets much stronger, it also refines. Let's consider how the Bible does these things for our spirit.

Heat Brings Warmth and Comfort

What's so great about heat? We use heat to relax our muscles when we've strained them. We're soothed by being wrapped in a warm blanket and snuggled close. We associate warmth with love and acceptance ("She's got a wonderful warmth about her") while someone who's uncaring is described as "cold." Stories that comfort us are described as "heartwarming," while news that upsets us is "chilling." When we come in to stand by a crackling fire in the fireplace after being outside in the freezing cold, we feel secure and relieved.

Our world is a cold place. Daily we hear of bombings, shootings, sudden deaths, unexplained sickness, famine, and cruelty. And on a smaller scale, there are stresses and frustrations that splash cold water on our daily lives. When we don't know where to turn for comfort during tough times, we become chilled. Where can we find comfort and warmth?

I'm sad to say that many people turn to false sources of heat for comfort. We've become a society that finds more authority in the opinions of celebrities than in the Creator of the universe. We tend to fill up on advice from talk shows instead of the advice of God. If someone is famous enough to have a show, make a movie or an album, or shoot a basketball accurately, we expect these people to offer guidance and answers.

The Bible tells us of our real source of strength:

My comfort in my suffering is this: Your promise preserves my life. The arrogant mock me without restraint, but I do not turn from your law. I remember your ancient laws, O LORD, and I find comfort in them. (Psalm 119:50-52)

May your unfailing love be my comfort, according to your promise
to your servant. (Psalm 119:76)

Let's take comfort from God's Word instead of huddling around false
sources and telling ourselves we feel warm when we're actually freezing our
spirit.

Heat Refines for Purity

It's by intense heat that metals are refined and any impurities are removed.
Metals such as gold and silver are heated until they're fiery hot, and
through the process, they become pure. Let's look at what the Bible says
about this use of heat:

- *God's Word is as perfect as highly refined silver.* The psalmist wrote,
  "And the words of the LORD are flawless, like silver refined in a
  furnace of clay, purified seven times" (12:6). We can trust the
  Bible as the pure Word of God. Think of drinking the purest
  water or eating the finest foods. We want to fill our bodies with
  incredible goodness like that, and our hearts deserve nothing less
  than the purest message.

- *God uses times of trial to test and refine us.* Again in Psalms we
  read, "For you, O God, tested us; you refined us like silver"
  (66:10). And the book of Isaiah says, "See, I have refined you,
  though not as silver; I have tested you in the furnace of affliction"
  (48:10). The Bible lets us know that God uses our difficult times
  to make us more pure. I imagine God is trying to burn off all the
  fats in our spirit and let them melt away. What's left is the best
  and the strongest part of us to serve him.

- *God's Word leads us to purity.* The psalmist asked, "How can a young man keep his way pure?" Then he provided the answer: "By living according to your word" (119:9). It is the cleansing blood of Jesus that purifies our hearts—no amount of clean living will do that. But living according to God's Word keeps our hearts pure once we've been washed by Jesus. When we follow the principles and commands of the Bible, we stay clean and unmarred by sin.

AN INEXHAUSTIBLE ENERGY SUPPLY

Light also provides energy. We were reminded about the energy that comes through photosynthesis, and we can think of other ways light provides energy as well. Have you seen homes or other buildings with solar panels on the top or side to capture energy from the sun? Scientists and inventors have harnessed the sun's energy for all kinds of uses. Likewise, the Bible gives us energy by providing the power, strength, and courage we need to stay spiritually strong.

Power Source

We see a great example of the power of the Scriptures when Jesus was alone in the wilderness. He hadn't eaten for forty days, so you can imagine he must have been *really* hungry. Along came the devil to tempt Jesus with food in order to gain control over him. Satan said, "If you are the Son of God, tell these stones to become bread" (Matthew 4:3).

Jesus had the ability. Jesus had the hunger. He must have been physically weak from lack of food, and I know when I'm physically weak I'm more susceptible to temptation. Maybe Jesus was feeling this way too. But instead of giving in to Satan, he found strength and power to fight back...in the Scriptures.

"Man does not live on bread alone but on every word that comes from the mouth of the LORD," he replied, quoting from Deuteronomy 8:3. The devil then began using Scripture in his own attack. Twice more Jesus answered the devil with words of God, using them for strength when he was weak.

How often are we tempted, not just by chocolate pie or potato chips, but by lust, anger, gossip, jealousy, and all those other nasty fats that entice us to take an unholy path? How can we manage to turn away from evil thoughts and actions? Where do we get the energy to fight back? What's our source of power? Yes, the Bible. If Jesus could use it to fight the devil, so can we.

Psalm 119:11 reflects, "I have hidden your word in my heart that I might not sin against you." This verse makes a great case for Scripture memorization—or at least having a firm grasp of biblical principles. If we don't have God's Word in our hearts, we don't have a ready defense against evil.

A New Testament verse, Ephesians 6:17, echoes this theme. Talking about spiritual armor, the apostle Paul tells us to take up "the sword of the Spirit, which is the word of God." This powerful weapon gives us energy to fight the fats that can bombard our spirit.

Strength and Courage to Carry On

There are countless stories of Christians who have been persecuted and martyred for their faith. Persecution continues today in much of the world and yet Christians persevere. I can't imagine the pain some men, women, and even children endure for the name of Jesus Christ. How do they do it? They receive power from the Holy Spirit, and they receive strength and courage from the Bible.

Thankfully, most of us will never endure severe persecution, but we still need strength and courage. What about the courage to tell your next-door neighbor that Jesus loves him? What about the strength to go to work each day when your coworkers fill your ears with gossip? What about the perseverance to make it through another day when your spirit is overcome with sadness or even depression? How do we do it? The Bible reminds us that God is with us in those times when we're lacking courage:

Be strong and courageous. Do not be afraid or discouraged because of the king of Assyria and the vast army with him, for there is a greater power with us than with him. (2 Chronicles 32:7)

My soul is weary with sorrow; strengthen me according to your word. (Psalm 119:28)

Because of my chains, most of the brothers in the Lord have been encouraged to speak the word of God more courageously and fearlessly. (Philippians 1:14)

Throughout the Bible, men and women were asked to trust God with their lives, and God gave them courage through his presence. When we read of these people, we're reminded that we serve the same powerful God, and he will provide for us in the same way. Even when courage is not specifically mentioned, we find people who received it and whose stories can encourage us: Noah, as he built the ark; Ruth, as she moved to a strange country with her mother-in-law; Esther, as she stood up for her people in the face of death; the disciples and early Christians, as they faced torture, imprisonment, and death. The history of our faith as recorded in the Bible is a great source of energy and courage for us.

START FILLING UP

You may be thinking that you're not a pro at studying the Bible or that you just don't find it all that interesting. Here are some ideas to get you started on filling up your spirit through God's Word:

- Set aside a short amount of time each day and read only for that period. Start with ten minutes, and simply read as much as you can. You don't have to read a whole book of the Bible, or even one chapter, with each sitting.

- Choose a book of the Bible that interests you. Many of the Old Testament books read like adventure or love stories. Genesis and the first part of Exodus, Joshua, Judges, Ruth, and Esther contain many heroic events and proof of God's faithfulness. In the New Testament, read John or Acts to rediscover God's powerful love for us.

- Your mother probably told you never to write in books, but make an exception with your Bible! Spend a month highlighting in one color words and phrases that reveal who God is. Then choose another color and highlight words that help you under-stand a specific issue such as joy or faith. Jot notes to yourself in the margin, telling how a verse has touched your life or what it means to you. Then as you revisit these sections over the years, you'll be reminded of the insights you received—and you'll be able to see your growth over time.

- Try reading a different version of the Bible. Most people have trouble reading the *King James Version* with its *thee*s and *thou*s. Try a paraphrase or a newer version and see if it helps you get a better grasp on the meanings of the words.

- Join a Bible study group. Learn from others who perhaps have studied more deeply than you have, and share what you're learning with others.

- Pick up a Bible study guide from your pastor, church library, or local Christian bookstore. Many practical guides are available that can lead you step by step through the books of the Bible or topics for Christian growth.

There are many ways to fill up on the Bible. If you read Deuteronomy fifteen years ago and gave up on the Bible after that experience, pick it up and try again! Give your spirit the light it needs. Fill up! Start today!

THIRTEEN

Filling Up on God's Family

And let us consider how we may spur one another on toward love and good deeds. Let us not give up meeting together, as some are in the habit of doing, but let us encourage one another—and all the more as you see the Day approaching.

—HEBREWS 10:24-25

My dad is an avid gardener. As far back as I can remember, he's always had a vegetable garden with tomatoes, spinach, corn, beans, and squash. When the corn was ready, Dad would have Mom boil water, then he'd quickly pick the corn, shuck it, and pop it right into the hot water. Within a few minutes, we'd be sinking our teeth into the fresh and tender kernels. Ahhh. Even now my dad manages to grow flowers and vegetables in the desert land of Arizona, daily nurturing his plants till they are lush and beautiful.

I like to think that I've inherited a few good traits from my father, but I'll be quick to admit that a green thumb is not one of them. I vow each spring to have a lush lawn, aromatic flowers, and more vegetables than our family could possibly eat. And each year I end up with a patchy lawn, a few marigolds, and a lot of rhubarb. (It's the only thing that seems to grow no matter how much I neglect it!) I've come to accept the fact that I'm not a good gardener.

Plants need water and light, as we've seen, but they also need to be tended. They need gardeners who will cultivate them. In order to grow and mature in our faith, we need the same thing. We need people who will care for us and encourage us. We need people who will nurture our spirit. Where can we find "gardeners of the spirit" who can help us grow? The best place is the church—a body of fellow believers who will nurture us, help us spot and remove weeds, and help us bear fruit.

THE CHURCH

Before we look at specific ways Christians can help each other grow, let's clarify a few things. First, when we talk here about church, we're not talking about a building. Many of us go to church on Sunday or other days of the week. Yet we can be inside that building day after day and never become a part of the church body that meets there. When we talk about church, we're talking about the assembly of Christians who form a community.

Second, I understand that different churches have different beliefs, different forms of leadership, and different traditions. It can get downright confusing! But as the Bible describes this assembly of believers, we are given a number of clear instructions as to what a church—*any* Christ-following church of any denomination in any part of the world—is to be. We'll focus on these clear instructions.

Third, churches can unintentionally thwart our efforts to achieve a Low-Fat Lifestyle. We're encouraged to serve others, which God instructs (see Galatians 5:13). But we can become like Martha, the friend of Jesus who focused so much on getting a job done that she failed to simply sit at the feet of Jesus and enjoy his presence. There are many opportunities to be involved in our churches, and we should find ways to serve and learn. But remember to choose the *best* from among all the good opportunities. In earlier chapters we learned that less is more, and this principle holds true when cultivating a rich spiritual life. It's wise to choose a few activities that afford a deep, meaningful experience.

Finally, while plants cannot tend to each other, Christians *do* tend to each other within the church. So as you benefit from fellowship with others in your church community, others also benefit from fellowship with you. Over the years, I've heard countless people say, "I don't need to go to church. I can read my Bible and pray at home and I do just fine." Yes, we can grow on our own, but those who follow this "Lone Ranger" approach are missing out on one of God's greatest blessings. They don't benefit from the nurture of others, and just as important, they never have the opportunity to help others grow.

WE ALL NEED TO BE NURTURED

My neighbor tends to her garden as if it were a part-time job. She's always out there pulling weeds, pruning, watering, and moving plants to places where they'll get more sun. With the nurture her plants receive, they're sure to thrive.

That's the picture I get when I think about my church involvement. I love to go to church and be nurtured! When I walk through those doors, I know people will water my spirit by leading me in worshiping God through song and prayer. Others will shine sunlight onto my heart by teaching me from the Bible and challenging me to look deeper into my spirit. And there will be those who gather around me and pray for the concerns in my life. These things happen to me on Sundays, and they also happen throughout the week as I talk to people from my church over the phone, over lunch, and at formal or informal prayer gatherings.

When we're part of a Christian community, we'll also have people around us who will help identify and pull out the weeds that are choking us. Weeding is a way to nurture a plant, and it's a way believers can nurture each other as well. Like fats, weeds take up too much space and don't leave room for what's good.

I have a friend I'll call Tamara, who grew up in a Christian home but later turned away from God and made some poor decisions. This past year Tamara felt God's pull on her heart and became a part of our church community. Being around other Christians who are caring for her, Tamara is growing in her faith. But there is a "weed" in Tamara's life, a sin habit that she recognizes but is unwilling to let go. Those of us who know Tamara love her even though we are sad about her choice.

Tamara came to me recently and asked if she could help lead our children's ministry. She's warm, caring, and thoughtful, and would make an ideal leader—except for this sin habit. I told Tamara I would love to have her involved as a leader, but that this "weed" in her life would not be a good example to the kids. It's a hard thing to say to someone, but I had to lovingly tell Tamara that she needed to pull this sin out of her life before she could be a leader.

Tamara wants to grow, yet this weed chokes her growth. Yes, she can grow to some extent, but as long as she holds on to this sin habit she will always feel hindered in her relationship with God. Something is blocking her from all the water and sunlight that she needs. And she is also being choked from receiving the blessing of leading others in their growth.

Some people are great at locating the weeds in the lives of others but have a hard time seeing the ones in their own lives. Jesus reminded us of this when he said,

> Why do you look at the speck of sawdust in your brother's eye
> and pay no attention to the plank in your own eye? How can you
> say to your brother, "Brother, let me take the speck out of your
> eye," when you yourself fail to see the plank in your own eye?
> You hypocrite, first take the plank out of your eye, and then you
> will see clearly to remove the speck from your brother's eye.
> (Luke 6:41-42)

So if we are doing some weeding in someone else's life, we need to be sure the dandelions and crabgrass aren't choking us, too.

How are you being nurtured by other Christians? Are you filling up on the worship and teaching being offered? Are you looking for ways to nurture others with your words and actions? And what about those weeds? Are you being honest with others and letting them help you pull the weeds that steal the nutrients from your spirit? These things won't happen by accident—it's up to you to take action!

MUTUAL SUPPORT

I have tall metal cages that are made to support tomato plants. The idea is that tomato plants get so big and the fruit so heavy that they need support to maintain their growth. I've rarely managed to have tomato plants grow to the point where they need support, so I've considered tying streamers to my metal cages and turning them into a sort of lawn art. But in the meantime, I keep them around with hopes that my plants will one day need help bearing their load.

The church is where we can find help in bearing our load. We're reminded of this responsibility in Galatians 6:2: "Carry each other's burdens, and in this way you will fulfill the law of Christ." Romans 12:10-13 speaks of the devotion we can show to each other through our care:

> Be devoted to one another in brotherly love. Honor one another above yourselves. Never be lacking in zeal, but keep your spiritual fervor, serving the Lord. Be joyful in hope, patient in affliction, faithful in prayer. Share with God's people who are in need. Practice hospitality.

Let me tell you about one of the remarkable examples I've recently seen of Christians living out these passages. At the center of the story is a woman in our church I'll call Janet, who had great difficulty controlling her anger. As a result she lashed out at a crying infant who was in her care, shaking the child in her frustration. Tragically, the child was blinded, and Janet must serve a number of years in prison. She knows what she did was wrong and lives with the load of guilt as well as the grief of being kept away from her husband and daughters.

The fourth-graders in our church were learning about God's love and forgiveness, and they decided to show these qualities to a member of our body who needed them most. They chose Janet. This group of children began writing letters to her, telling her they were praying for her. They sent her small gifts such as stamps and handmade cards. Then they asked the other children in our congregation to contribute money, which was given to Janet's family to assist with gasoline costs on their long drives to the prison for visits. These children then collected money for the family of the little boy who had been blinded.

The gifts of these children are small in some ways. They cannot give Janet her freedom. They cannot restore sight to the baby boy. Yet they help to bear the load, to support the hurting. These young Christians have lived out the words of Ephesians 4:32: "Be kind and compassionate to one another, forgiving each other, just as in Christ God forgave you." They are already learning how to support others in the body of Christ.

I cannot count the times I've both taken meals to families in need and received meals when we were in need, the times I have been called on to help and the times I have called out for help. Over and over again, I've seen Christians support each other. It's so encouraging to bring up this topic with other Christians and hear about the times they've been supported when the load was too much to bear—and to hear the joy in their voices as they tell about the times they've been able to help others. What a privilege we have!

AN EXTRA MEASURE OF NUTRIENTS

Sometimes plants need a little extra boost. They've had water and sunshine, the soil has been turned, the weeds pulled. The plants may be growing but they're not thriving. They may need a little fertilizer, an extra dose of nutrients. For Christians, this kind of boost comes in the form of encouragement and fellowship.

Can you think of a time when someone has encouraged you and really made a difference in your life? I know there have been times in my life when I've been reading God's Word, worshiping, and praying, yet still I have felt discouraged. Then I open the mail and find a card from a friend. It makes me smile or laugh, and my spirit gets a boost. What's more, I've found that when I try to encourage someone else, I feel encouraged myself. It's contagious! The Bible tells us of the importance of encouraging each other:

> Therefore encourage one another and build each other up, just as in fact you are doing. (1 Thessalonians 5:11)

> But encourage one another daily, as long as it is called Today, so that none of you may be hardened by sin's deceitfulness. (Hebrews 3:13)

> And let us consider how we may spur one another on toward love and good deeds. (Hebrews 10:24)

When we encourage others, we're building them up—just what our spirit needs to grow! Encouragement keeps our hearts from being hardened by sin. And I love the thought of being spurred on toward love and good actions. As a part of God's church, find a way you can encourage someone else today—and every day this week. Try a few of these ideas:

- Take flowers to someone.
- Write a note. Share a funny story or a meaningful verse.
- Call someone just to see how he or she is doing. A lot of people say, "No one ever calls me." Do you call them?
- Leave an anonymous gift on someone's doorstep. Ring the doorbell and run!
- Invite someone out for coffee or frozen yogurt.
- Mail a card. Say, "This made me think of you."

- Offer to baby-sit so a friend can have a night off.
- Give a hug. Even squeezing a hand works.
- Tell a friend about a song that reminds you of him or her.
- Invite a friend to run errands with you—it's fun to be included.

Another way to give nutrients to the spirit is through fellowship. Some churches serve red punch and cookies and call this "The Fellowship Hour." I'm sure some fellowship takes place there, but that doesn't have to be all there is. Find ways to go deeper so you truly become a part of a community. In my own life I experience fellowship on several levels. On Sunday morning I see many people, greet them, and chat for a few minutes. That's a light touch of fellowship. Then on Thursday nights, Mike and I get together with a group of about ten couples. We share what's happening in our lives and pray for each other. We laugh a lot, cry a bit, and do what we can to support and encourage each other. That's fellowship on a deeper level. And twice a month I have lunch with three other women. I can share even more deeply and honestly with these women. I know what I say will be kept in confidence, and I know these dear friends will pray for me and hold me accountable for my actions. It's fellowship on an even deeper level.

Where are you finding fellowship? It may start with the light fellowship of greeting and shaking hands on a Sunday morning, but it needs to go deeper than that. Otherwise no one will ever know your needs or know how to encourage your spiritual growth. And you won't know how to meet the needs of others.

Some people go into a church and say, "No one talked to me. No one was friendly. I'm not going back." Friendliness and fellowship are two-way streets. Remember that a lot of people are just as uncomfortable as you are in taking the initiative to offer a handshake and a word of kindness. So don't put a burden on them. Make the first contact, and make an acquaintance who might turn into a friend. Look for places you can get involved and find deep fellowship.

BEARING FRUIT

When we garden, we want to see good results. We want our flowers to bloom, and we want to see fruits and vegetables ripen and mature so we can enjoy eating them. A Christian spirit that has been watered in worship and prayer, that has basked in the sunlight of God's Word, and has been tended by loving Christians will bear fruit as well. Galatians 5:22-23 tells us what the result of steady growth will be: "The fruit of the Spirit is love, joy, peace, patience, kindness, goodness, faithfulness, gentleness and self-control. Against such things there is no law."

Are these qualities apparent in your life? These are the evidence that your spirit is growing and that you've cut out the fats of bitterness, hate, jealousy, anger, and even spiritual lethargy, making room for God's beautiful fruit of the Spirit to bloom in your heart. These are the proof that you've got a low-fat spirit.

The other evidence shows in how you use your spiritual gifts. In 1 Corinthians 12:12-26, the apostle Paul gives a picturesque illustration of how we are to work together in serving God and each other. This passage compares the body of Christ to a physical body. So I might be a liver, you might be a toe, and another might be a knee. Each body part has a purpose, and to live without one of them can be difficult and painful, even life-threatening in some cases. We need all our body parts to work together for the health and effectiveness of the body.

That's how God envisions us as Christians—working together in harmony and interdependence to accomplish his goals for us.

Ephesians 4:16 says, "From him the whole body, joined and held together by every supporting ligament, grows and builds itself up in love, as each part does its work." Without each of us doing our part, others may not grow. And if others don't grow, we might not grow either. We depend on one another in our church communities. It's part of the low-fat spirit. Cut out attitudes that keep you from using your gifts and enjoying the gifts of others. Fill up on what God has poured into your spirit, then make use of it.

Body, Soul, and Spirit

I have come that they may have life, and have it to the full.

—JOHN 10:10

Body. Soul. Spirit.

We've covered them all. We've discovered how to make our creed a reality. We can honestly say, *Daily I will fill my life with an abundance of that which is healthy so that I will no longer need—or eventually even want—that which is unhealthy.*

We know what's healthy for our bodies and how to fill up on those things. We know how to select the foods that fill us with nutrition, not fat.

We know what's healthy for our souls, for our daily lives, and how to fill up on those things. We know how to choose the attitudes and activities that will not fill our days with stress and frustration.

We know what's healthy for our spirit and how to fill up on those things. We know how to cleanse our hearts of the fats that lead us to depression, anger, hate, and sadness. We know how to fill up on God's grace and love.

I hope along the way you've been taking action: evaluating your eating habits, your daily activities, your spiritual being, and making choices that will let you fill up on God's goodness and leave behind what's unnecessary for your life. There's a lot to consider, and some choices aren't easy to make. With God's help, you can do it! Life is too short to not live it to the fullest.

Remember the promise Jesus made: "I have come that they may have life, and have it to the full" (John 10:10). That is our ambition—to experience all the fullness and goodness life has to offer. As we replace the fats in every aspect of our lives, we will be filled up with the joy and contentment that come only from God.

Notes

Chapter 1

1. "U.S. Warning of Death Toll from Obesity," *New York Times,*
   14 December 2001. Found at www.nytimes.com/2001/12/14/health/
   14OBES.html.

2. "Is Total Fat Consumption Really Decreasing?" *Nutrition Insights, A Publi-*
   cation of the USDA Center for Nutrition Policy and Promotion, April 1998.

3. "Beliefs and Attitudes of Americans Toward Their Diet," *Nutrition Insights,*
   A Publication of the USDA Center for Nutrition Policy and Promotion, June
   2000.

4. Dean Ornish, *Eat More, Weigh Less* (New York: HarperCollins, 1993), 6.

5. Ornish, *Eat More, Weigh Less,* 6. See also "Low-Fat Living: How Much Fat
   Is Okay?" found at www1.xe.net/lowfat/articles and "Avoiding the Fat-Free
   Trap" by Lisa Stollman, M.A., R.D., C.D.E., found at www.heartinfo.org.

6. Ornish, *Eat More, Weigh Less,* 20.

7. "Pass the Pork Rinds, Consumers Want the Fat," *Loveland Daily Reporter-*
   Herald, 25 June 2001, sec. B-4.

8. Adapted from several height and weight charts, including: 1983 Metro-
   politan Life Insurance Height and Weight Tables (www.parkinson.org/
   nt6.htm), Heartscreen (www.heartscreen.com/hw_info.html),
   Arnot Ogden Medical Center (www.aomc.org/HOD2/general/
   weight-Height_W.html), and several others.

9. This chart was created using the mathematical formula discussed in this
   chapter.

Chapter 2

1. Thomas B. Costain, *The Three Edwards* (New York: Doubleday, 1958), 179-80.

2. Robert Pritikin, quoted in Gary Smalley, *Food and Love* (Wheaton, Ill.: Tyndale, 2001), 59.

3. George Will, "Make That Supersized, Please," *Loveland Daily Reporter-Herald,* 27 February 2002, sec. A-4.

4. Dean Ornish, *Eat More, Weigh Less* (New York: HarperCollins, 1993), 61.

5. Smalley, *Food and Love,* 8.

Chapter 3

1. Gary Smalley, *Food and Love* (Wheaton, Ill.: Tyndale, 2001), 19-20.

Chapter 4

1. "Menu Maneuvers," *Cooking Light.* Found at www.cookinglight.com.

2. Eric Schlosser, *Fast Food Nation* (New York: HarperCollins, 2002), 3.

3. Paula Kurtzweil, "Today's Special: Nutrition Information," U.S. Food and Drug Administration. Found at www.fda.gov/fdac/features/1997/497_menu.html.

4. Schlosser, *Fast Food Nation,* 3.

5. Schlosser, *Fast Food Nation,* 6.

6. George Will, "Make That Supersized, Please," *Loveland Daily Reporter-Herald,* 27 February 2002, sec. A-4.

7. Mary Duenwald, "An 'Eat More' Message for Fattened America," *New York Times,* 19 February 2002. Found at www.nytimes.com.

8. Duenwald, "An 'Eat More' Message."

9.   "Waistlines Victim of Value Marketing," *Loveland Daily Reporter-Herald,* 11 March 2002, sec. A-4.

10. Schlosser, *Fast Food Nation,* 66.

11. Kurtzweil, "Today's Special: Nutrition Information."

12. Jayne Hurley and Stephen Schmidt, "Chinese Food: A Wok on the Wild Side," *Nutrition Action Health Letter,* September 1993. Found at www. nutritionaction.org/nah/chinese.html.

Chapter 6

1.   To read the original account of this story, see 1 Samuel 17.

2.   Mike Nappa, *The Courage to Be Christian* (West Monroe, La.: Howard, 2001), 83.

Chapter 7

1.   Rabbi Marc Gellman and Monsignor Tom Hartman, "How Do You Find God?" *Reader's Digest,* April 2002, 98.

2.   James Dobson, *Stories of the Heart and Home* (Nashville, Tenn.: Word, 2000), 235.

3.   All three quotes are from promotional materials for David Hazard, *Reducing Stress* (Eugene, Oreg.: Harvest House, 2002).

Chapter 9

1.   Suze Orman, *The Courage to Be Rich* (New York: Riverhead, 1999), 36.

2.   Orman, *The Courage to Be Rich,* 3.

3.   "Debt Statistics" from Neway. Found at www.neway.org/debtStatistics.html.

4.   Robert G. Allen, *Multiple Streams of Income* (New York: John Wiley & Sons, 2000), 25-6.

5. From Merriam-Webster Web site, www.m-w.com.

6. This happened to a missionary supported by our church—for obvious reasons, I don't want to give names!

Chapter 10

1. This story and quotations are from the Women with Vision Conference, April 27-28, 2001, where Jill Briscoe was the keynote speaker.

2. Chip Dodd, *The Voice of the Heart: A Call to Full Living* (Franklin, Tenn.: Providence House, 2001), 10.

Chapter 11

1. Thomas Aquinas, quoted in Edythe Draper, *Draper's Quotations for the Christian World* (Wheaton, Ill.: Tyndale, 1992). From the *QuickVerse 5.0* CD-ROM by Parsons Technology.

2. Matt Redman, *The Unquenchable Worshipper* (Ventura, Calif.: Regal, 2001), 25.

3. Charles Swindoll, quoted in Draper, *Draper's Quotations for the Christian World.*

Chapter 12

1. Bruce Olson, *Bruchko* (Coral Springs, Fla.: Creation House, 1978), 137-43.

2. "Photosynthesis," *Microsoft Encarta Online Encyclopedia 2001.* Found at encarta.msn.com (23 April 2002).

Recommended Resources

Part 1: The Low-Fat Body

Eat More, Weigh Less by Dean Ornish, M.D., Spotlight Publishing—This book
provides advice from a medical expert with studies and research to back
it up.

Fast Food Nation by Eric Schlosser, Perennial Publishing—This is an exposé
about fast-food restaurants, filled with facts and stories that may change the
way you eat.

Food and Love by Dr. Gary Smalley, Tyndale House Publishers—This book
explores the connection between our emotions and our eating habits.

www.PictureTrail.com/doktordi by Dr. Diane Komp, host—This Web site provides
recipes for many delicious and easy-to-prepare dishes.

Part 2: The Low-Fat Soul

Reducing Stress: Natural Remedies for Better Living by David Hazard, Harvest House
Publishers—This book looks at what stress does to our lives and then gives
sensible advice on how to lower stress permanently.

Pictures Your Heart Remembers by John Trent, Ph.D., WaterBrook Press—This
offers a touching look at the impact our choices make in dealing with negative
memories.

Simplify Your Life and Get More Out of It! by H. Norman Wright, Tyndale House
Publishers—The author offers practical ideas on getting rid of clutter in all
areas of life.

Other Resources

Lower the clutter in your life by cutting down on the junk mail you receive. Have your name taken off mail sales and marketing lists by sending a letter with your name, address, and phone number to:

Mail Preference Service

c/o Direct Marketing Association

P.O. Box 9008

Farmingdale, NY 11735-9008

Lower the fat of phone sales calls. Have your name taken off telephone sales and telemarketing lists by sending a letter with your name, address, and phone number to:

Telephone Preference Service

c/o Direct Marketing Association

P.O. Box 9014

Farmingdale, NY 11735-9014

Part 3: The Low-Fat Spirit

A Woman's Touch: The Fingerprints You Leave Behind by Amy Nappa, Howard
    Publishing—This book explores the ways God has touched your heart and
    how you pass that touch on to others.

The Courage to Be Christian by Mike Nappa, Howard Publishing—This is a
    challenging book with many insights into spiritual growth.

FAQ: Frequently Asked Questions About the Christian Life by Ray Pritchard,
    Broadman & Holman Publishers—The author covers the basics of the
    Christian faith with insight and wisdom.

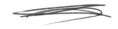

⚡LIFE IN THE⚡
THIRD REICH

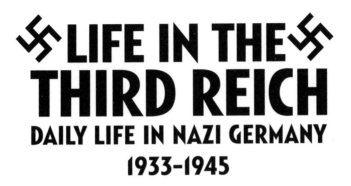

LIFE IN THE THIRD REICH

DAILY LIFE IN NAZI GERMANY

1933–1945

PAUL ROLAND

ARCTURUS

ARCTURUS

This edition published in 2016 by Arcturus Publishing Limited
26/27 Bickels Yard, 151–153 Bermondsey Street,
London SE1 3HA

Typesetting by Palimpsest Book Production Limited
Cover image: courtesy of Bundesarchiv/Bild-146-1973-060-021/
o.Ang

ISBN: 978-1-78599-019-9
DA004560UK

Printed in China

Contents

Preface

When the Allies occupied a defeated Germany in the spring
of 1945 they shared a desire to mete out retribution to those
members of the Nazi leadership and their minions who had
brought so much suffering and destruction to the world
during five long years of war. This need was felt particularly
strongly by the Russians, who believed that they had suffered
the most from the barbarous cruelty handed out by Hitler's
forces in their crusade to subjugate the Slavic people and
eradicate the blight of communism from Eastern Europe.

The problem was that it was not so easy to identify the
middle- and lower-ranking Nazis once they had divested
themselves of their uniforms, destroyed all incriminating
documents and melted into the chaos of a disintegrated
society. In the ensuing confusion, justice was rough and
ready, frequently dispensed without due process by battle-
weary, sleep-deprived soldiers who were understandably
unforgiving and disinclined to adhere to the Geneva
Convention. It was not unknown for captured Nazi officers
who calmly enquired where they would be billeted to be

deliberately pointed in the direction of patrols with instructions to shoot enemy soldiers on sight.

Senior Allied officers had devised their own way of distinguishing Nazi sympathizers from the general population. They were confident that if they were approached by civilian officials eager to assure their liberators that they had not been loyal Nazis, the officers could be sure they had identified the very Nazis they were looking for and could promptly lock them up.

Although Hitler, Himmler and Goebbels had all committed suicide in the final days of the war and many senior-ranking SS officers had evaded justice via the so-called 'Vatican rat lines' to South America, the Allies had some success in delivering formal justice to those they held responsible for

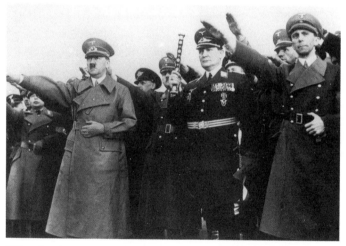

Hitler, Goering and Goebbels and other high profile members of the Nazi leadership were familiar faces through newsreels and newspapers but other members of the regime would prove hard to identify and track down.

'waging aggressive war' and for initiating 'crimes against humanity'. They put 22 of the most notorious members of the Nazi leadership on public trial at Nuremberg in November 1945, among them Hermann Goering, Rudolf Hess, Joachim von Ribbentrop and Albert Speer. Martin Bormann, Hitler's private secretary, was tried and found guilty in absentia. His fate was the subject of much speculation for almost three decades until his remains were discovered not far from Hitler's Berlin bunker in 1972 and formally identified using genetic testing in 1998. The 23rd defendant, Robert Ley, had taken his own life before the trial began.

Behind closed doors, the judicial process had been fraught with unseemly squabbling between the Soviets and their former allies, who disagreed on many significant details. Overall, however, there was a belief that justice had been done and, more importantly, had been seen to be done. By the time subsequent trials had taken place of senior Nazi judges, members of the SS, a dozen or so extermination camp doctors and the most sadistic female concentration camp guards, the will to prosecute a vanquished enemy had given way to the desire to make the best of the peace that had been hard won and at such an enormous cost. Those Germans living in the west of their divided country were now allies of the European democracies, who were engaged in a Cold War with the Communist Bloc. The Soviet presence in East Germany and particularly in a partitioned Berlin was seen as a real and immediate threat to world peace. Consequently, Nazi hunting was left to amateurs such as Simon Wiesenthal, a Holocaust survivor who would not let the world forget that men such as Dr Josef Mengele and Adolf Eichmann were still at large.

Servicemen and women were impatient to go home and get on with their lives, and there was a general need to leave the horrors of the war in the past. Besides, there was a serious danger in presuming collective guilt when even the de-Nazification courts had identified three levels of 'offenders', distinguishing between the leadership, who would be indicted for 'waging aggressive war', and their subordinates accused of war crimes – as distinct from those deemed to be mere 'followers', who were unlikely to face prosecution. The process of de-Nazification was considered so large and complex that General Eisenhower estimated that it could take 50 years to purge Germany of Nazi ideology.

However, Germany's infrastructure and administration was in ruins, so pragmatism and realpolitik took precedence. In 1945, eight and a half million people – more than 10 per cent of the population – were still registered members of the Nazi party, with the highest proportion being civil servants, lawyers and teachers. As these individuals were needed to run basic services, their past was frequently overlooked. In the 1950s, it was estimated that 60 per cent of the civil servants in Bavaria were known to be former Nazis, but it was not until the 1960s that the next generation began asking awkward questions of their parents and querying the complacency of Konrad Adenauer's government regarding the prosecution of war criminals in the immediate post-war years.

The fact of the matter is that Hitler's Germany was not comprised of hard-core fanatics, with a small minority actively or passively opposed to the regime (the latter justifying their failure to act by citing the feeble defence known as 'internal emigration', a term coined by German writer Erich Kastner).

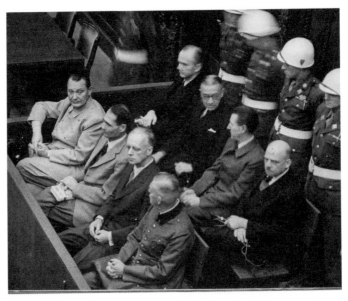

The defendants in the dock at Nuremberg, November 1945. Of the 22 former functionaries of the Nazi leadership on trial, only Goering retained any semblance of his once formidable personality.

Even among the most devout followers, there were those who 'had their reasons' for being converted to the Nazi cause. Fifteen-year-old Hilde Schlegel joined after attending an event organized by the party at which she tasted real buttered rolls for the first time and consequently believed that Hitler would ensure a better quality of life for the underprivileged. Some joined out of self-interest, seeking advancement; others for the reasons frequently cited by historians – the belief that the National Socialists would bring political stability, prosperity, employment and the return of territory seized under the hated Versailles Treaty.

But as this book will show, a sizeable proportion of Germany's citizens impassively witnessed the country's descent into dictatorship because they believed they were simply powerless to prevent it – as well as many more who could not see the danger until it was too late.

Chapter One
The Worst of Times

The Aftermath of 1918

'The confused locksmith Drexler provided the kernel, the drunken poet Eckart some of the "spiritual" foundation, the economic crank Feder what passed as an ideology, the homosexual Roehm the support of the Army and the war veterans, but it was now the former tramp, Adolf Hitler, not quite thirty-one and utterly unknown, who took the lead in building up what had been no more than a back-room debating society into what would soon become a formidable political party.'

(William L. Shirer on Hitler's takeover of the German Worker's Party in 1921)

The Nazis did not attract their initial supporters through persuasive political argument, nor by appealing to their ideals and aspirations, but by simply promising to provide for their immediate and fundamental needs – work and bread. Many who voted for them in the 1920s and even some of those who joined their ranks and marched under their banners during these early days of 'the struggle', sincerely and naively believed that National Socialism offered the only credible opposition to Bolshevism.

Not all of Hitler's early followers shared his virulent anti-Semitism, or subscribed to the more fanciful elements of his party's pseudo-völkisch ideology, which declared that the Germans were descendants of an Aryan master race and were destined to rule over inferior nations.

In the immediate aftermath of the country's defeat of November 1918, the population was weary, dispirited and looking for a leader with ready answers – someone who could identify those who were to blame for their misfortunes.

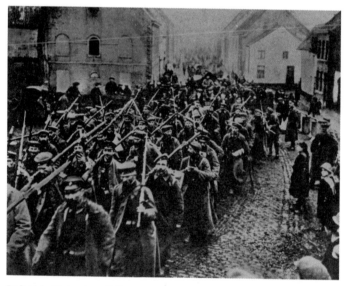

Defeat in November 1918 was seen as more than a military debacle. It brought humiliation to the German soldier who soon subscribed to the myth that the Army had been 'stabbed in the back' by defeatism generated at home by weak, defeatist politicians.

Families throughout the country were grieving for the incalculable loss of life, confounded by the sudden and unexpected capitulation of an army they had been assured was on the verge of victory, and embittered by the futility of the sacrifice they had made in vain for the Fatherland. This sense of despair was compounded by the abdication of the Kaiser and the new Weimar government's willing compliance with the punitive terms and conditions imposed by the Versailles Treaty. It is therefore no wonder that this poisonous atmosphere gave rise to extreme nationalism and the belief that the army had been betrayed, or 'stabbed in the back', to borrow a phrase attributed to General Ludendorff.

This grievous wound might have healed over time had it not been aggravated by the rampant inflation of 1922–3, which saw savings wiped out and wages devalued to the point where workers were being paid twice a day so that they could buy food while it was still affordable. Even so, it was not uncommon to see customers paying for produce with what had once been a month's wages, all of which emphasized the fragility of the economy and the ineffectiveness of the Weimar government. Within a year the average price of a loaf of bread had risen from 165 marks to one and a half million.

In every village, town and city, men, women and children could be seen begging for food and spare change, or asking for menial work of any kind. Into this desperate situation the Nazis appeared under the guise of the National Socialist German Workers' Party with a promise of jobs for the unemployed and relief for the impoverished. In addition, they declared their intention to purge commercial institutions of Jewish influence and to rid German business of 'unfair competition' (i.e. Jews). They vowed to crush the communists and put an end to the frequent and bloody skirmishes between rival political factions that made the streets unsafe for law-abiding citizens. They would also restore national pride by tearing up the hated Versailles Treaty and demanding the return of territory seized by the Allies after 1918. Every citizen was persuaded to believe it was his or her patriotic duty to vote for the programme. Hitler's critics accused him of being a crude, ill-educated rabble-rouser, but he articulated the people's anger and sense of injustice more effectively than the professional politicians and it was evident that he had touched a raw nerve.

'He was not easily discouraged. And he knew how to wait. As he picked up the threads of his life in the little two-room apartment on the top floor of 41 Thierschstrasse in Munich during the winter months of 1925 and then, when summer came, in various inns on the Obersalzberg above Berchtesgaden, the contemplation of the misfortunes of the immediate past and the eclipse of the present, served only to strengthen his resolve ... And there was born in him anew a burning sense of mission – for himself and for Germany – from which all doubts were excluded.'

(William L. Shirer on Hitler after his release from Landsberg Prison in December 1924, having served 264 days for planning the failed Munich Putsch [coup] the previous year.)

The Nazis' popularity rose and fell during the 1920s as the economy recovered then dipped again following the 1929 Wall Street Crash. But by 1933, the German people had lost their patience with their elected representatives and were prepared to set aside any concerns they might have had with

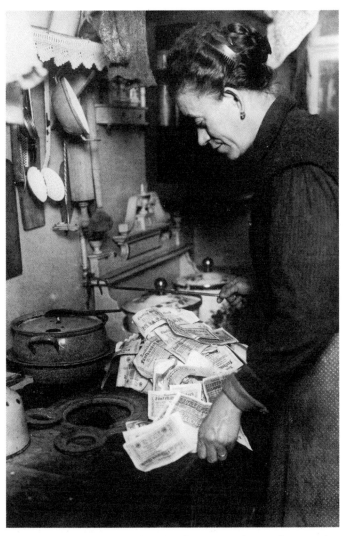

When inflation was at its height the German mark was of more value as fuel for the kitchen stove than as currency.

regard to the reported 'excesses' of the SA (the party's brown-shirted enforcers) to give these untested newcomers a chance.

However, there was nothing inevitable about the Nazis' seizure of power. In the final parliamentary election before Hitler was handed the chancellorship by the ageing President Hindenburg in January 1933, the party suffered a significant reversal of fortunes. Its share of the vote fell from 37 per cent to 33, giving it fewer than 200 seats in the Reichstag – just a third of the total. But Hitler's acolytes were certain that it was only a matter of time before their day would come.

First Signs

'As the year of 1931 ran its uneasy course, with five million wage earners out of work, the middle classes facing ruin, the farmers unable to meet their mortgage payments, the Parliament paralyzed, the government floundering, the eighty-four-year-old president fast sinking into the befuddlement of senility, a confidence mounted in the breasts of the Nazis.'

(William L. Shirer, *The Rise and Fall of the Third Reich: A History of Nazi Germany*)

For Berlin schoolboy Bernt Engelmann, the first indication that there was something distinctly sinister lurking behind the men in the brown shirts who had been pamphleteering and making street corner speeches in his neighbourhood came on a Monday morning in May 1932. It would be eight months before Hitler became chancellor, but already there were visible signs that his followers were impatient for power. Someone had hoisted a large swastika flag from the roof of the secondary school in Wilmersdorf and it was attracting the attention of students and staff. One of the teachers ordered the janitor to take it down, but the man just grinned insolently and protested that he didn't have the key to the turret door. Several older students laughed at this and one remarked that if the hoisting of the flag was a sign that Hitler was already in power, then 'heads would roll', a notion that appeared to please the janitor.

Incensed, the teacher strode off to inform the principal, who was already on the phone protesting to the superintendent of schools, but before any action could be taken another teacher was seen to emerge from an upper window, clamber onto the roof with the nimbleness of a mountaineer and tear down the flag. This was greeted with much encouragement from the boys who had gathered in the yard and whose spontaneous applause drowned out the boos and hisses issued by their Nazi-loving classmates. The feat was all the more remarkable as it had been accomplished by the French master, Dr Levy, who had lost an arm in the Great War. But if the boys expected to be regaled with details of Dr Levy's exploits during that morning's class they were to be disappointed. Even after he had slid the blackboard up to write on a second slate panel underneath and had found the words *Salope Juif!* [Jewish Sow] scrawled in large letters, he remained calm and composed. He simply explained that the phrase showed an incorrect use of French grammar and that the more appropriate phrase was *Manchot Juif*, meaning a Jewish veteran.

Engelmann estimated that of the 450 pupils in his school about 40 had expressed Nazi sympathies. That morning they were inflamed with victory, the party having just won a

majority in the regional election in Oldenburg, and the
despised Chancellor Brüning had resigned. It would be only a
matter of hours, they believed, until President Hindenburg
appointed Hitler his successor. They would not take the
insult of having their flag removed without a fight. During
recess, three of the older boys marched into the principal's
office to register a complaint against Dr Levy – two bore the
uniform of the Hitler Youth and the third was in SA brown
shirt, breeches and boots in defiance of a government ban on
the wearing of paramilitary uniforms. Instead of calling the
police, the principal placated them by promising to suspend
Dr Levy until a full investigation could be held.

His capitulation was perceived by the Nazi bullies as
permission to take their spite out on the Jewish students.
Several ganged up on the younger boys, whom they beat
mercilessly with their fists and belts until they bled.
Engelmann witnessed several such incidents that morning.
But the Nazis were not yet in power and there were still
sufficient numbers of outraged parents to question the principal's handling of the affair. For all his talk of proceeding
with 'utmost severity' against those seeking to politicize the
school, Engelmann's parents had detected a note of
sympathy in his voice towards the Nazis. It was just one
example of what the American oral historian Studs Terkel
called a lack of 'civil courage' and it could be argued that
this form of cowardice was as much to blame for the rise
of Hitler as the uncritical adoration heaped upon him by
his supporters.

Not long after this incident, the Engelmann family
moved to Düsseldorf, where Bernt attended a school that
had not yet been infected by what he describes as the
'contagion of Nazi ideology'. He attributed his instinctive

revulsion for rabid nationalism to the environment in which he grew up. His father was a staunch believer in democracy, his mother had offered practical assistance to the 'victims of an obviously inhuman policy' and his grandfather, a trade unionist, Social Democrat and confirmed pacifist, had advised the boy to join a Socialist Workers' youth group. Bernt's paternal grandmother also instilled in him a distrust of sabre-rattling militarism and the conservative aristocracy who, she said, regarded the top government posts as their birthright. But it was only when Bernt witnessed the public burning of books written by authors that he had read and admired that he realized the Nazis were the enemies of educated, free-thinking people such as himself.

Later, as a young man during the war, he joined a resistance group but was arrested by the Gestapo and interned in Flossenbürg and Dachau concentration camps. After Germany's capitulation, he became an eminent investigative journalist and returned to Berlin, where he interviewed many of the people with whom he'd grown up during the 1930s. He was shocked to discover that several of his former friends had highly selective memories of that period and that more than a few attributed their participation in the Hitler Youth to nothing more than 'youthful idealism'.

There was Marga, for example, a pretty, vivacious girl who recalled the thrill of the street parades with their flags and bunting and singing in the streets. She told him, 'All in all, we had a wonderful carefree youth, didn't we?'

Marga's father, a presiding judge of the district court and an ardent Nazi, had forbidden his wife from shopping at Jewish-owned stores and had been strict with their daughter, insisting that she be home every evening by 7 pm. But after the *Röhm Putsch* [the 'Night of the Long Knives'] on 30 June 1934, he had been a changed man. The news that Hitler had ordered the murder of more than 1,000 people without trial (some of whom were silenced to prevent them revealing details of his past) had left the judge disillusioned and seriously questioning his allegiance to the party. He no longer objected to his wife shopping at Jewish-owned stores. Nor did he seem to care what time his daughter came home. It appears that one of his friends, the music critic Dr Wilhelm Schmid, had been murdered on the Night of the Long Knives by four SS men, who had dragged him from his apartment and shot him in the mistaken belief that he was the SA leader Willi Schmidt.

Marga hadn't thought to ask her father or mother why her father had changed and it was only two years later, after she had married, that he spoke about it.

All Marga could recall were the popular songs of the time, the balls she had attended and the films she had seen. She remembered the first time she and Bernt had been to the theatre to see a performance of Friedrich Schiller's *Don Carlos* and could still recall the names of the cast, but she had no idea why members of the audience had broken into spontaneous applause during a scene in which one of the characters implores his employer, 'Sire, grant us freedom of thought', until Bernt explained it had been to demonstrate their opposition to the regime's suppression of free speech.

It was experiences such as these that led Engelmann to conclude that the Nazification of his country was neither the work of 'sinister demons' nor the inevitable result of 'grim fate' for which no one could be held accountable, but simple self-interest and timidity.

Hearts and Minds

The Nazis had made a concerted effort to win over the hearts and minds of the population, ingratiating themselves with every section of German society and making promises they had no intention of keeping. They had also mastered the art of political propaganda by staging mass rallies and marches that emphasized their unity and fanaticism but which gave a false impression of their popularity. Their campaign to win the state of Lippe in the January 1933 parliamentary election was typical.

Unless they won this marginal state and made up for the serious reverses they had suffered throughout the country in the November 1932 Reichstag elections, it was feared that the industrialists and bankers would withdraw their financial support and the party would give in to factional infighting and eventually destroy itself. Consequently, Hitler and Goebbels mounted a sustained campaign using the last reserves of party funds and every publicity stunt they could conceive of to secure the votes of the 100,000 inhabitants.

Over ten days they staged 900 events, with Hitler delivering speeches at 16 major rallies. Thousands of SA and SS men were drafted in to march through the streets of every town and village in the region, shouting slogans and putting on a show of strength while cars equipped with loudspeakers urged the population to vote. It created the impression that the party was not only substantial and well funded but also very popular. In fact, despite all of their parades and pageantry, they managed to increase their share of the vote by only 6,000.

The democratic parties won a total of 50,000 votes between them to the Nazis' 39,000, but the right-wing ultra-nationalist press hailed it as a significant victory and a fortnight later President Hindenburg was persuaded to appoint Hitler the new chancellor.

A Better Class of People

'In the summer of 1933 ... any collective resistance had become impossible; individual resistance was merely another form of suicide.'
(Sebastien Haffner, quoted in *German Voices* by Professor Frederic C. Tubach)

Horst Kruger, the teenage son of a Berlin civil servant, witnessed the euphoria that greeted Hitler's accession to the chancellorship in 1933:

'It was a cold night in January and there was a torchlight parade. The radio announcer, whose resonant tones were closer to singing and sobbing than reporting, was experiencing ineffable events ... something about Germany's reawakening, and always adding as a refrain that now everything, everything would be different and better ... The time was ripe ... a surge of greatness seemed to course through our country...'

That week it looked as if every house and business in the quiet suburb of Eichkamp had hung out swastika flags and even children's bicycles were adorned with a fluttering pennant, many of them handmade by the parents because the manufacturers couldn't cope with the demand. Horst's parents had not shared their friends and neighbours'

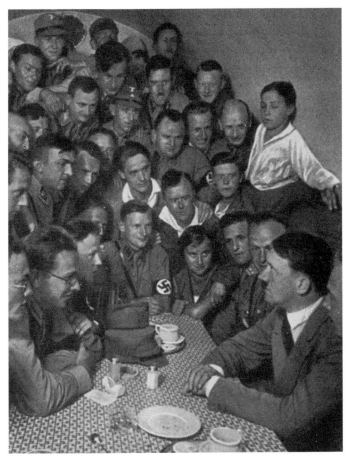

The Führer became the centre of a personality cult, which saw him mobbed by adoring followers at his many carefully stage-managed personal appearances.

enthusiasm for the new administration, but they were quietly hopeful that it signalled an end to the economic uncertainty that had hung over the country in the past few years and that it might stop the outbursts of violence between rival political groups. So they joined in with the celebrations, if only to show their willingness to give the Nazis a go and also to demonstrate their good will and sense of community.

'Suddenly one was a somebody,' Horst recalled, 'part of a better class of people, on a higher level – a German.'

Everybody was included. At least everyone who was an ethnic German. But even many Jews hoped that the anti-Semitic frenzy they had suffered might die down now that the party was in power and that its extreme elements might be reined in, if only to quell criticism in the foreign press. Private anxieties were put on hold for the duration while the country turned out en masse for what seemed at the time to be a series of endless parades and processions. The jubilant atmosphere was heightened with the announcement of new holidays celebrating various aspects of German life and culture, and when the extensive programme of public works was announced, the excitement escalated. The misery of crip-pling unemployment and economic depression appeared to have been erased at a stroke. People were buoyant, optimistic and alive with a sense of purpose. Members of the Labour Service marched through the streets with spades slung over their shoulders on their way to lay the foundations for a new Germany that would be connected by an extensive network of autobahns. But after the new art galleries and government ministries had been built on a grand scale, the rundown tenements and slums remained and the same people who had waved their flags and cheered the processions consoled themselves with the thought that Hitler could not work miracles overnight. They would have to be patient.

And when it was announced that the SA had been purged of its more unruly elements in order to supress a counter-revolution, these same voices asked themselves if Hitler could have known about it and that, even if he had, he would surely not have approved of such barbarity.

Horst recalls that his neighbours were galvanized with a sense of national pride and excited at the prospect of being part of a more productive and prosperous nation. Bierkellers were packed with men holding forth on every aspect of government policy, from the reclaiming of territory occupied by the Allies to the benefits of the autobahn. They were under the impression that they would have a say in both international and local affairs, and soon became 'disarmed, willing and docile', consenting to anything the new administration cared to ask them to endorse through the ballot box. While the men boasted of standing up to the League of Nations as if it were a disagreeable neighbour, their wives discussed the possibility of having or adopting children to fulfil their maternal duty to the Fatherland.

With each new territorial acquisition, Hitler's reputation as a statesman increased tenfold. To have achieved such significant and substantial gains without embroiling the country in a war and in the face of international condemnation seemed to confirm that the Führer had been sent by God to reclaim what was Germany's by right. His ardent admirers began to snip his speeches out of the newspapers so they could discuss them with their family and friends as they might once have debated the Sunday sermon. Horst's mother was typical, he says, of those who 'lived on

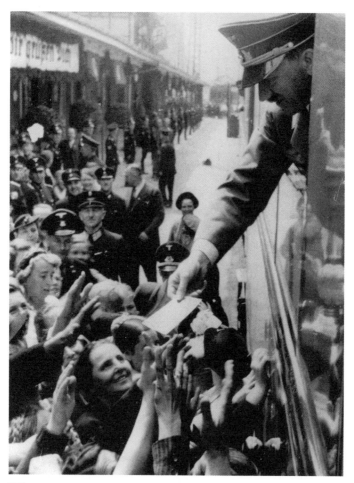

Hitler was venerated throughout the Reich as a saviour sent by God to restore national pride and recover territory occupied by the victorious allies after the First World War.

illusions'. A devout Catholic, she saw Hitler as the penniless artist who had risen above his lowly origins to restore Germany to its rightful place on the world stage and whose faith would inspire him to make the well-being of the people his priority. The Führer, she assured her son, would not lie to his people.

Horst considered his neighbours to be 'honest believers, enthusiasts, inebriates' who had convinced themselves that life would be better under Hitler and who hoped that talk of war was no more than malicious rumours. Hitler did not want war, they told themselves – but when it came, many realized that Hitler had not only conquered Europe, he had also subjugated his own people. They existed merely to serve him.

Nazification

The administration's first proclamation was drafted to reassure the people of its reactionary credentials.

'The new national government will consider its first and supreme duty to restore our nation's unity of will and spirit. It will safeguard and defend the foundation on which the strength of our nation rests. It will firmly protect Christianity, the basis of our entire morality, it will safeguard the family ... It wants to base the education of Germany's youth on a reverence for our great past, on pride in our old traditions. It will thus declare war on spiritual, political and cultural nihilism ... the government will once again make national discipline our guide.'

(Adolf Hitler, 1 February 1933)

The Nazi leadership sought to cultivate an image of themselves as the architects of a new classless society in which employers were expected to take their meals with their employees and professionals worked side by side with the unqualified in state-regulated organizations such as the Labour Front. They also advocated unrestricted access to the universities and military academies for loyal party members, something that had previously been a privilege enjoyed only by the aristocracy and ruling elite. A limit was introduced, however, for female students enrolling in university, amounting to no more than 10 per cent of the total.

Hitler had prohibited women from taking an active role in politics and the professions, although he permitted them to work as unpaid activists drumming up support for the party and caring for its underprivileged members. Their natural place in the National Socialist state was to be selfless mothers of blond, blue-eyed Aryan babies, a role encapsulated in the party slogan *Kinder, Küche und Kirche* [Children, Kitchen and Church].

'The National Socialist revolution,' Hitler proclaimed, 'would be an entirely male event.' Nevertheless, 34,000 middle-class, middle-aged housewives had joined the party by 1933 – women such as Gertrud Scholtz-Klink, nominal figurehead of the Nazi Women's Union, whose fanatical loyalty earned her the nickname 'the Female Führer'; Elsbeth Zander, founder of the Order of the Red Swastika; Elizabeth Polster, who increased the membership of the National Socialist Women's Organization (NSF) by persuading her 66,500 members that Christianity and National Socialism were not mutually exclusive; and Guida Diehl, whose Nationalist Newland Movement predated the founding of the Nazi party by five years.

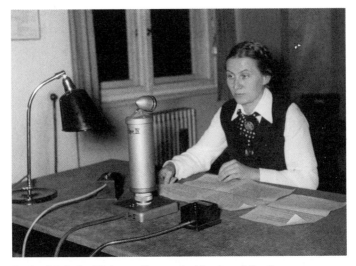

Gertrud Scholtz-Klink was the nominal leader of the German Women's Union, which claimed to have more than 6 million devoted followers but had no influence on policy. She was known as 'The Female Führer'.

As for unmarried single women, they were regarded as second-class citizens or *Staatsangehöriger* [subjects of the state], and afforded the same legal status as Jews and mentally disabled people. And yet, a significant proportion of Hitler's most ardent supporters were women, although it is a myth that they voted in greater numbers for the Nazis than for rival parties.

In practice, Hitler's inner circle paid only lip service to the principles of National Socialism. In private, Goebbels, Goering and their cohorts indulged to excess in their magnificent private villas while their wives flaunted their Paris fashions and cosmetics in defiance of their Führer, who had declared such luxuries to be ostentatious, vulgar and unpatriotic. Only Frau Bormann cultivated the dowdy peasant look that her Führer considered to be the image of the ideal German mother. She dressed in Tracht [heritage clothing] as dictated by the Reich Fashion Institute, braided her hair in a bun and declined to wear lipstick in the belief that it was made from animal fat, as Hitler had stated. Every year for ten years she dutifully bore another child.

Devoted to the Cause

Those who volunteered for local party activities invariably found that there was scant reward or acknowledgement for all the time and energy that they had devoted to the cause.

Typically, members of the Nazi Women's League would be put to work collecting dues and contributions to party funds, applying to various offices and agencies responsible for housing large families whom the party had promised to help; later they would assist with rehousing those who had been bombed out of their homes. Every free moment they could spare would be devoted to party projects of one sort or another and their only recognition would be a front seat at various local events, or perhaps the honour of presenting a bouquet to party officials, maybe even the Führer himself. These women, by all accounts, rarely complained and also remained staunchly loyal even after they were forced to face the horrors perpetrated by the regime.

More often than not they would blame Heinrich Himmler or other Nazi leaders but rarely Hitler, whom they believed shared their concern for the welfare of the German people. They dismissed the rumours regarding the extermination camps and atrocities committed by the SS in the conquered territories as malicious gossip. At party meetings they swallowed the official line – that the concentration camps had been built to imprison criminals, profiteers and other undesirable individuals who would be taught discipline and re-educated. The newspapers regularly reported details of those who had been arrested and what crime they had committed against the state to merit their subsequent internment, or execution. This made a mockery of their claim after the war that they knew nothing of what took place at camps within Germany, such as Dachau near Munich and Ravensbrück, north of Berlin. Such measures were generally considered necessary and it was understood that the inmates deserved to be dealt with severely. To enforce the impression that only habitual offenders were imprisoned in camps within Germany, the press printed photographs of individuals specially selected for their 'repulsive' appearance.

It was in the regime's interest to publicize the existence of the camps to act as a deterrent and this gave rise to the saying, 'Hush! Watch out! You don't want to end up in a concentration camp.'

Alignment

It was shortly after Hitler's appointment to the chancellorship that the new administration implemented the policy they called *Gleichschaltung* [bringing into line], which forced all institutions and various aspects of social and political life to conform to and adopt Nazi ideology. It began with a clampdown on Catholic youth organizations, the banning of Catholic publications, the closure of Catholic hospitals and schools and the imprisonment of the clergy, accused of decadence by Nazi publications such as *Der Stürmer* and *Das Schwarze Korps*. The regime also outlawed the Catholic Centre Party along with all opposition parties and removed many Catholics from civil-service posts.

Even high school students were obliged to sign a declaration of allegiance to the new regime in 1933. Helene Jacobs refused and was consequently barred from taking her final exams. On leaving school she found poorly paid employment with a Jewish attorney, but believing that the Nazis would soon be forced out of office she was determined to stick to her principles. She considered the whole idea of an Aryan master race to be contrary to everything that she had been taught and was determined to express her disapproval:

> *'The point that aroused me from the beginning was that we as a people had to show our unwillingness in some fashion, not just when the crimes began, but before, when it started, with this so-called "Aryan" ancestry. They distributed questionnaires and you had to say whether you had "Aryan" ancestors. Everyone filled them out. I said, "We can't go along with this; it's not legal. We must do something against this and throw the questionnaires away." But today – the other people my age, they behaved totally differently at that time. Most of them built their careers then. When I said, "I'm not going to have anything to do with this," I isolated myself.'*

(Victoria Barnett, *For the Soul of the People*)

Gleichschaltung was not confined to state schools. Universities too were infiltrated by the New Order's enforcers.

Peter Drucker, a Frankfurt University lecturer, hoped that he might be able to remain in his post but was shocked by what he witnessed during the first Nazified faculty meeting held just weeks after Hitler had become chancellor:

'Frankfurt was the first university the Nazis tackled, precisely because it was the most self-confidently liberal of major German universities, with a faculty that prided itself on its allegiance to scholarship, freedom of conscience and democracy. The Nazis therefore knew that control of Frankfurt University would mean control of German academia. And so did everyone at the university. Above all, Frankfurt had a science faculty distinguished both by its scholarship and by its liberal convictions; and outstanding among the Frankfurt scientists was a biochemist–physiologist of Nobel-Prize calibre and impeccable liberal credentials.'

Drucker had never thought it necessary to attend a faculty meeting, but when a Nazi commissar for Frankfurt was appointed in the spring of 1933, he hoped that his pronouncements would provoke a reaction from the faculty members that would force the Nazis to back down and respect the university's autonomy.

'The new Nazi commissar wasted no time on the ameni-
ties. He immediately announced that Jews would be
forbidden to enter university premises and would be
dismissed without salary on March 15; this was something
no one had thought possible despite the Nazis' loud
anti-Semitism. Then he launched into a tirade of abuse,
filth, and four-letter words such as had been heard rarely

*even in the barracks and never before in academia. He
pointed his finger at one department chairman after
another and said, "You either do what I tell you or we'll
put you into a concentration camp." There was silence
when he finished; everybody waited for the distinguished
biochemist–physiologist. The great liberal got up, cleared
his throat, and said, "Very interesting, Mr Commissar, and
in some respects very illuminating: but one point I didn't
get too clearly. Will there be more money for research in
physiology?" The meeting broke up shortly thereafter with
the commissar assuring the scholars that indeed there
would be plenty of money for "racially pure science". A
few of the professors had the courage to walk out with
their Jewish colleagues, but most kept a safe distance
from these men who only a few hours earlier had been
their close friends. I went out sick unto death – and
I knew that I was going to leave Germany within
forty-eight hours.'*

An anonymous college professor excused his support for
the New Order in a conversation with American academic
Milton Mayer after the war by explaining that he had
been swept along by the surge of enthusiasm for the new
administration and what promised to be a new era of study
and scholarship.

*'Middle High German was my life. It was all I cared about.
I was a scholar, a specialist. Then, suddenly, I was plunged
into all the new activity, as the university was drawn into
the new situation; meetings, conferences, interviews,
ceremonies, and, above all, papers to be filled out, reports,
bibliographies, lists, questionnaires. And on top of that were*

demands in the community, the things in which one had to, was "expected to" participate, that had not been there or had not been important before. It was all rigmarole, of course, but it consumed all one's energies, coming on top of the work one really wanted to do. You can see how easy it was, then, not to think about fundamental things. One had no time. Too Busy to Think.'

The professor admitted that the new routine, the continuous changes and crisis engineered by the regime:

'... provided an excuse not to think for people who did not want to think anyway ... Most of us did not want to think about fundamental things and never had. There was no need to.'

The ever-present threat posed by enemies within and without distracted 'decent' people from considering the consequences of what they were participating in, until it was too late to do anything.

'Suddenly it all comes down, all at once. You see what you are, what you have done, or, more accurately, what you haven't done (for that was all that was required of most of us: that we do nothing). You remember those early meetings of your department in the university when, if one had stood, others would have stood, perhaps, but no one stood. A small matter, a matter of hiring this man or that, and you hired this one rather than that. You remember everything now, and your heart breaks. Too late. You are compromised beyond repair.'

(Milton Mayer, *They Thought They were Free*)

Working Under the Nazis

But the Nazis did not manage to intimidate everyone. Less fanatical party members might overlook critical remarks said in their presence by friends, while some even went so far as to warn communist colleagues of an imminent wave of arrests. This was especially true among manual workers in the factories, shipyards and on the railways, where comradeship often came before party loyalty. The suspect could then lie low for a few days and their absence could be blamed on a bout of illness. But many political opponents of the regime were not so fortunate. Anyone could be sacked on the spot without reason, although the official pretext for their dismissal would be put down to 'political unreliability'.

Skilled workers tended to be better informed about their rights and valued their unions, which the Nazis abolished as soon as they seized power. These men felt aggrieved that the regime now forbade them any say in working conditions and excluded them from wage negotiations. They resented the fact that Hitler had established Labour Trustees and that he had authorized these to set wages that were often agreed behind closed doors with management.

Manual labourers and white-collar workers were also acutely aware that their wages declined steadily during the Nazi era, while income from factory ownership and investment rose. Workers found themselves putting in longer hours and working faster to meet production targets in the hope of receiving an increase in wages.

While the Nazi leadership declared their solidarity with the people, they enacted laws that bound workers to a form of medieval serfdom. Under the Law for the

Organization of National Labour (passed in 1934), for example, industry regressed to a feudal system with employees reduced to the status of servants. If an employer didn't want an employee to leave, they could refuse to hand over the documents that were required whenever someone began a new job.

The regime attempted to appease the workers and get the most out of them by initiating a programme they called *Kraft durch Freude* [strength through joy], which offered incentives to productivity in the form of holidays and state-subsidized leisure activities. By 1937, almost 38.5 million Germans had participated in these state-sponsored leisure activities, which included symphony concerts, theatre performances, cruises to Scandinavia and Spain and breaks to the German countryside.

It all sounded too good to be true and it was. The beneficiaries of these bonuses were often the highly skilled workers, administrative staff and management.

One branch of Robert Ley's organization promoted the building of leisure facilities and canteens in factories and offices, which employees were shocked to learn they would have to build and pay for themselves.

But the most cynical strategy was the offer of a Volkswagen car, which workers paid for over several years but that was never produced. Every employee who signed up for the scheme had 5 marks a month deducted from his or her wage packet in addition to taxes and compulsory contributions to Nazi welfare organizations. After three-quarters of the price had been paid, the employee would receive a voucher with an order number. They were never told, however, that the factory built to assemble the cars had been converted for the production of munitions.

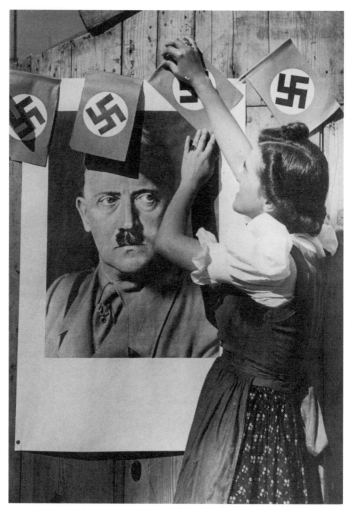

Nazism insinuated itself into every aspect of its citizens' lives. This was not a burden for those who believed that life would get better under Hitler's leadership.

Undermining the Family

*'The National Reich Church of Germany categorically claims
the exclusive right and the exclusive power
to control all churches within the borders of the Reich:
it declares these to be national churches of the
German Reich.'*

(William L. Shirer, *The Nightmare Years*)

A more subtle and insidious tactic was for the regime to portray itself as the people's protector and benefactor, while at the same time usurping parental influence and undermining the authority of organized religion.

This process was formalized by the Enabling Act passed just one week after the burning of the Reichstag on 27 February 1933 – which is generally believed to have been planned and executed by the Nazis, who needed a pretext to persuade President Hindenburg to pass an emergency decree suspending civil rights. The act was blamed on a lone Dutch communist with learning difficulties, Marinus van der Lubbe, who was tried and summarily executed after a show trial. He was the first of 12,000 civilians to be eliminated by Nazi 'special courts' during the Third Reich (see: Peter Hoffmann, *The History of the German Resistance 1933–1945*).

Once the dictatorship had tightened its stranglehold on all government administrative offices and public institutions, it sought to insinuate itself in every aspect of its citizens' public and private lives. In May 1933 all trade unions were abolished and workers' rights were regulated by the Labour Front. The family was infected by Nazi ideology, which indoctrinated children, turning them against their parents, and attempts were made to supplant religion with a neo-pagan form of worship that deified Hitler as the saviour of the nation.

Hitler repeatedly stressed the role Christianity would play in the National Socialist state while at the same time promoting specious Nazi ideology that was in direct contradiction of Church doctrine. It required that marriages and funerals be formalized as neo-pagan ceremonies, with the swastika replacing the crucifix on the altar, the Bible substituted by *Mein Kampf* and prayers replaced with an oath of allegiance to the head of state.

For a time, many regular churchgoers couldn't understand why their pastors were censuring the new administration in their weekly sermons when conditions had improved significantly for the average working family. But then the book burnings began, followed by concerted attempts to challenge the authority of the Church and its clerics' objections to the systematic elimination of those individuals who were deemed to be of no value to the state.

Book Burning

On 10 May 1933, students in Berlin and other major German cities organized the public burning of books deemed to be 'un-German'. These included titles by Thomas Mann, H. G. Wells, Jack London, Sigmund Freud, Albert Einstein and the blind American author and political activist Helen Keller. Propaganda minister Josef Goebbels had incited the students of Berlin with a rabble-rousing speech that betrayed the real reason for this act of intellectual vandalism: the Nazis feared anything that encouraged the masses to think for themselves and to question the validity of whatever they were told:

> *'...The era of extreme Jewish intellectualism is now at an end ... The future German man will not just be a man of books, but a man of character. It is to this end that we want to educate you. As a young person, to already have the courage to face the pitiless glare, to overcome the fear of death, and to regain respect for death – this is the task of this young generation. And thus you do well in this midnight hour to commit to the flames the evil spirit of the past. This is a strong, great and symbolic deed...'*

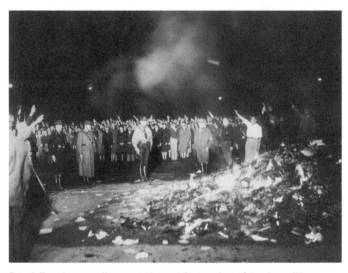

Bernt Engelmann witnessed the public burning of books written by authors that he had read and admired and realized that the Nazis were the enemies of educated, free-thinking people like himself. Nazism signalled not a political revolution but a return to barbarism.

The burnings provoked outrage around the world. Keller's book *How I Became a Socialist* was among the books hurled on the pyre. In an open letter to the student body of Germany, she expressed the ire and alarm that many artists and intellectuals felt on reading the reports of that night's events:

> *'History has taught you nothing if you think you can kill ideas. Tyrants have tried to do that often before, and the ideas have risen up in their might and destroyed them.*

> *'You can burn my books and the books of the best minds in Europe, but the ideas in them have seeped through a million channels and will continue to quicken other minds. I gave all the royalties of my books for all time to the German soldiers blinded in the World War with no thought in my heart but love and compassion for the German people.*

> *'I acknowledge the grievous complications that have led to your intolerance; all the more do I deplore the injustice and unwisdom of passing on to unborn generations the stigma of your deeds.'*

A hundred years earlier the German–Jewish poet Heinrich Heine had written, 'Where one burns books, human beings will inevitably follow.'

Chapter Two
The New Order

Myth of the Economic Miracle

*'The big businessmen, pleased with the new government
that was going to put the organized workers in their place
and leave management to run its businesses as it wished,
were asked to cough up. This they agreed to do at a
meeting on February 20 at Goering's Reichstag President's
Palace, at which Dr Schacht acted as host and Goering and
Hitler laid down the line to a couple of dozen of Germany's
leading magnates, including Krupp von Bohlen, who had
become an enthusiastic Nazi overnight, Bosch and Schnitzler
of I.G. Farben, and Voegler, head of the United Steel Works.
The record of this secret meeting has been preserved.'*
(William L. Shirer, *The Rise and Fall of the Third Reich: A History of
Nazi Germany*)

The population was indoctrinated with the lie that Hitler's
public works programme, such as the building of the
autobahn and the construction of the Siegfried Line (the
defensive line known by Germans as the Westwall), had
reduced unemployment, but it took the dictatorship almost

four years – until 1936 – to bring unemployment down to an acceptable level. By that time the other industrial nations had recovered from the Great Depression and had done so without drafting every able-bodied man into the army and their less able brethren into the munitions factories.

The 'economic miracle' that Hitler is credited with achieving in Germany was attained at considerable cost. The majority of men who were drafted in to build the autobahns had to live on wages that were lower than their unemployment benefit. They were paid 51 pfennigs an hour compared to 66 pfennigs for comparable work in a factory or printing shop and they were compelled to work in the open air regardless of the weather. To add to their misery, they were required to live far from home in barracks where the conditions were on a par with prison and for which

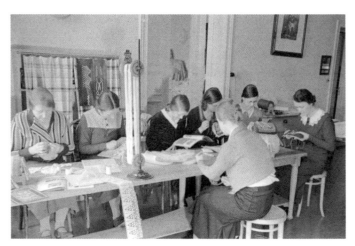

Women workers fared worse than their male colleagues and were typically paid a third less as well as having to pay for their own travel to a workplace chosen for them by the state.

they were required to pay 15 pfennigs a day plus another 35 pfennigs for slop ladled out of a cauldron. The average weekly wage for these manual labourers was 16 marks a week after these compulsory 'contributions' had been deducted and they were rewarded with just ten days' holiday per year.

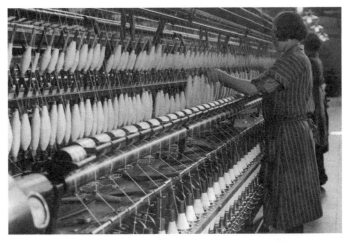

Many women were conscripted into factories and required to work 12-hour shifts.

Female workers fared even worse as they were not regarded as being of equal value. They were typically paid a third less than their male colleagues. A skilled female factory worker could expect to earn 35 marks a week with overtime, but from this she would have to deduct money for food supplied by the company and pay for her travel. Those who had been used to working a shift that allowed them to do their domestic chores before work now found themselves reporting to munitions factories or other branches of compulsory service as early as 6 am. If they lived far from the factory they would have to allow extra time for travelling, which meant that they could return home after a 12-hour shift to find most of the shops shut and those that remained open late with little fresh produce left to sell.

To add to their hardship, they would be too tired to take on the extra jobs such as office cleaning that might have earned them a few more marks a week. After paying for food and travel, many workers were left with just 10 marks a week. It was no wonder that the older women often suffered illness and fatigue, which increased dramatically with the onset of war, when Allied air raids frayed their nerves and deprived them of sleep.

Unemployment had been reduced from six million when Hitler came to power in 1933 to a third of that in just three years. However, the economy had suffered as a result because public works programmes had been financed by demanding that should banks issue massive loans, which wouldn't have been offered to a democratic government or private industry. The problem was compounded by the administration which printed the money required to pay for the loans. This would almost certainly have created hyperinflation had Germany not gone to war in 1939. But that had been Hitler's plan all along: he mobilized the population and increased the production of arms and munitions in order to wage war, not to create full employment or benefit the economy.

Shopkeepers and the owners of small businesses were another group who discovered that the party's election promises were no guarantee that their lot would improve under National Socialism. The Nazis had threatened to 'Aryanize' Jewish-owned department stores and firms that had been blamed for squeezing small traders and entrepreneurs out of business by buying in bulk and selling below the price their competitors could afford. But as soon as the Nazis had forced the Jewish businessmen out, they replaced them with Germans – some of whom proved even more ruthless when it came to cutting prices. The department stores remained open but under new German ownership and these men frequently refused to rent out units to small stallholders, something the previous owners had done. Many small businesses which had been holding out in the hope that the Nazis would create prosperity were forced to close, the victims of declining sales and customers who insisted on buying on credit because they couldn't pay outright for their goods.

Those whose shops and businesses struggled to remain profitable in the years before the war could appeal to their local *Kreisleiter* [block warden] to put in a word for them at local party headquarters, but frequently they were simply told to be patient, that Hitler couldn't perform miracles overnight and had to be given time for his economic programmes to take effect. When another year passed without any sign of improvement in trade, they might petition the *Kreisleiter* again, who would have been told by local party officials to advise the owners to sell out to the bigger stores or close their businesses and seek employment with the army. In the meantime, they could earn a little by selling subscriptions to the party newspaper, the *Völkischer Beobachter*, and collecting on behalf of the Winter Aid – although they themselves were probably in greater need of charity than the poor for whom they were collecting.

Hitler's Children

The basic facilities that we take for granted today were considered luxuries for many German working-class families in the 1920s and 1930s.

BDM [*Bund Deutscher Mädel*; League of German Girls] member Ursula Dickreuther remembered having to wash without hot water in their unheated city apartment block, even in the bitterest winter. Her family had to resort to filling hot water bottles and heating them on the stove to take the chill off their beds. If they were lucky, the water might still be lukewarm by the morning, when they would empty the contents into a basin to wash themselves.

There were communal bathrooms in most apartment blocks, so tenants had to take turns and agree on a rota with the other residents. Public bathhouses offered showers for 50 pfennigs or a bath for 1 mark, but the larger families would make do as best they could at home to save even a few marks. Bath day saw all of the children washed in the same wooden laundry tub, one after the other, with the youngest having the first dip and the eldest the last. All of them used the same water topped up with buckets of scalding-hot water heated on the stove. Dishes, too, were washed in water heated on the stove and afterwards the buckets had to be scrubbed with Vim to remove the grimy ring. Clothes were also washed by hand with a washboard and a hard bristle brush, but often only once a month, and the wet laundry would be hung up inside the apartment unless the weather was good. Laundry day was loathed by children as it was the day when their mother was too busy to make food, so they had to make do with soup and bread – if they could afford it.

As so many families were forced to share facilities it was

common to rely on chamber pots, which had to be emptied every morning. With no toilet paper, people were forced to use pieces of newspaper strung on a wire in the communal bathroom. Such hardship had its positive side, though. Ursula believes that it was her habit of reading these cuttings that gave her a head start with her education.

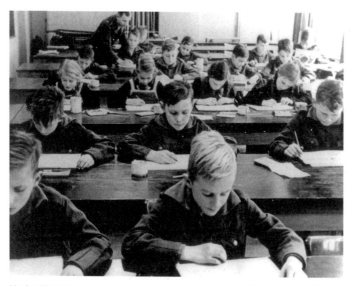

Under the Nazis, education became synonymous with indoctrination. Spurious racial theories were taught to children from the age of six and textbooks were liberally sprinkled with quotes from *Mein Kampf*.

Children born to working-class German families in the interwar years experienced much the same level of hardship as their equivalent in other European countries. They were expected to do their share of the chores, fetching coal and firewood, running errands, even sweeping, scrubbing and waxing floors, beating rugs and polishing brass door fittings until they could see their faces in them.

But when their tasks were done they could run freely in the streets, ride their bikes or scooters or have fun on roller skates, if they had any. All but the most basic toys and board games were too expensive for the average working family at that time, so children relied on popular street games that needed only a skipping rope, a ball or a piece of chalk. If they had none of these, then it was hide and seek, tag or cowboys and Indians.

Entertainment was limited to a rare trip to the circus, cinema, fair or theatre. Only the middle class could afford to go swimming in the municipal baths; everyone else had to wait for the warmer weather and make do with the local river or lake. But winter brought the excitement of sledging (you needed only a tray and some string to steer it with), ice skating (with or without skates) and of course snowball fights.

Euthanasia

For those suffering from a disability, life under the Nazis was to prove unspeakably cruel. It started when compulsory sterilization for blind, deaf and physically disabled people, and for those suffering from chronic depression, was legalized in 1933 with the passing of the Law for the Prevention of Hereditarily Diseased Offspring. Even chronic alcoholism was deemed to be sufficient grounds for treatment.

Two years later, the Law for the Protection of the Hereditary Health of the German People was enacted. This forbade German citizens with hereditary or infectious diseases from marrying and producing 'sick and asocial offspring' who would be expected to become a 'burden on the community'.

Over the following four years, 200,000 compulsory sterilizations were performed and an efficient system was put in place to implement the administration's euthanasia programme.

Gerda Bernhardt's mentally disabled brother Manfred was one of 5,000 children murdered by Nazi physicians on the Führer's whim. There was no official order as such, only a *Führerstaat* [directive] that had apparently originated with a casual remark made by Hitler to his personal physician, Dr Karl Brandt, concerning the merits of killing those 'unworthy of life'.

Gerda recalled:

'Manfred was a lovely boy, but he could only say "Mama" and "Papa" ... He only learnt to walk very late too. He always liked to be busy. If my mother said, "bring some coal up from the cellar", he wanted to do it over and over again. My father was in favour of putting him in some sort of children's hospital and then Aplerbeck came up as they had a big farm there and the boy might be kept occupied.'

Aplerbeck had been established as a 'Special Children's Unit' where patients would be given a lethal injection and their parents informed that they had died of natural causes.

Gerda recalls the last time she saw her brother alive. 'They brought the boy into the waiting room. There was an orderly there when I was leaving. The boy stood at the window and I waved and waved and he waved too. That was the last time I saw him.'

Indoctrinating the Young

Long before the Nazis came to power, Hitler had declared the education of Germany's children to be a priority, but after 1933, when state schools came under the control of the dictatorship, it became clear that it was not education that Hitler had in mind but indoctrination. Racial ideology and the spurious pseudo-sciences replaced traditional subjects such as biology and history.

Even maths was used to disseminate Nazi propaganda, with pupils being asked, for example, how many marriage loans of 1,000 marks could be paid out to worthy Aryan couples if the 300,000 mentally ill people in care at the cost of 4 marks a day could be eliminated. Teachers were required to sanction the new curriculum and to prove their loyalty to the party by joining the Nazi Teachers' Association – 97 per cent did so. The remainder were forced to leave their posts. One third of female teachers had been compelled to take early 'retirement' in the year Hitler came to power in order to fulfil their primary role as homemakers and mothers.

Both primary and secondary teachers were predominantly male and were required to attend political education classes and to refute their former political allegiances. But even after their training was completed, they were informed that their performance would be monitored by their own pupils. Any infringements, deviations or disloyal remarks would be reported to the Federal Ministry of Education, whose remit was to ensure that all schools, universities and research institutes conformed to National Socialist ideology.

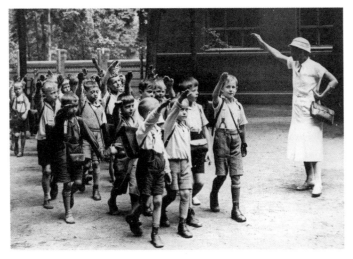

In *Mein Kampf* Hitler stated that the purpose of education was to prepare girls for motherhood and boys for the military.

A 1936/37 issue of Nazi women's magazine *Frauen Warte* itemized the educational principles of the New Germany:

> **Race**: National Socialist education means instruction in the ideas of the German people, in understanding German traditions, in arousing the pure, uncorrupted, and honourable people's consciousness, their sense of belonging to the community. Only an uncorrupted member of the German race can have such an understanding of his people, completing it with the willingness to sacrifice all for the nation.
>
> **Military training**: It is clear that the German youth must be determined to defend their Fatherland with their lives. Despite all the noise regarding promises and

disarmament, Germany is surrounded by enemies. The German youth must acquire military virtues. Their bodies must be hardened, made tough and strong, so that the youth may become efficient soldiers who are healthy, resilient, trained, vigorous and able to endure hardships.

Leadership: A youth being trained for such important national duties must accept the idea of following the Führer absolutely and without question, without damaging discontentment, criticism, without self-regard or resistance.

Religion: God and nation are the two foundations of the life of the individual and the community.

Although the German school system under the Nazis was designed to inhibit intellectual advancement and was geared to conditioning women to accept a submissive, secondary role in society, many of those who attended state schools during the Third Reich considered themselves to have been well educated.

The three-tier system of education that exists in Germany today was operating then. *Volksschule* catered for children from the ages of 7 until 11 and had segregated classes for boys and girls. At the end of the fourth year, pupils had the choice to stay on for another four years, after which they could leave full-time education without a qualification, or go on to a grammar school (high school) or a *Gymnasium* (comprehensive) for a further six years.

Both were exclusively for boys. If girls wanted to continue their education, their parents had to pay for them to attend a private school or *Lyceum*.

In secondary school, English was frequently taught as a

first foreign language with French as the second language. Boys might also be taught Latin. Grammar school girls would typically be taught secretarial skills, domestic science, needlework, art and music in addition to the basic subjects.

History was literally rewritten to emphasize the positive aspects of German nationalism and to apportion blame for the defeat of 1918 to the convenient scapegoats – the vindictive Allied victors and the Jews.

The subject of racial purity pervaded practically every subject from biology to geography, with an emphasis on the need for *Lebensraum* [living space for the German people]. The preservation of the 'superior' Aryan bloodline was emphasized and illustrated with insidious propaganda films comparing the Jews to plague-spreading vermin. These were enforced with film and photographs of mentally and physically disabled people to justify the state's policy of forced sterilization and euthanasia.

Fanciful racial theories were introduced to pupils from the age of six under the generic subject *Rassenkunde* [race knowledge] and were presented as proven fact of the superiority of the Aryan master race and the inferiority of the Jews and Slavic races. Students had no opportunity to question the validity of these theories as all Jews had been excluded from the public school system after 1935 under the Nuremberg Laws.

Older students also studied Philosophical Propadeutic (the history of philosophy), which had been introduced to instruct them in the specious unfounded beliefs of Nazi 'philosopher' Alfred Rosenberg, whose anti-Semitic diatribe *The Myth of the Twentieth Century* was the set text for the course. Its central argument was that man lacks a soul but is guided by intuition. According to Rosenberg, 'great men' such as Hitler were able to inspire their followers by appealing to their intuition, in the same way as religious leaders were believed to be able to raise the consciousness of their devotees and disciples. Hitler was said to have dismissed the book as pure gibberish, but it remained on the syllabus because it was marginally more comprehensible than *Mein Kampf*. In contrast, almost every textbook was peppered with quotes from the latter. Even a fifth-grade biology book for girls equated the hierarchy of the animal kingdom with the German nation's superiority and right to subjugate 'inferior' races:

'He who wants to live must fight, and he who does not want to fight in this world of perpetual struggle does not deserve to live!'

(Adolf Hitler, *Mein Kampf*)

And on the same page, the future mothers of the nation were reminded of their Führer's assertion that:

'The world does not exist for cowardly nations!'

It was also explicitly stated that the purpose of education was to prepare girls for motherhood and boys for the military:

'The goal of female education must be to prepare them for motherhood.'

(*Mein Kampf*)

'The task of the army in the ethnic state is not to train the individual in marching, but to serve as the highest school for education in service of the Fatherland.'

(*Mein Kampf*)

Physical fitness became a core subject in the curriculum; attendance was compulsory and ruthless competitiveness was rewarded. Failure to attain a minimum standard of fitness could result in expulsion, while exceeding the required standard might bring the pupil to the attention of the selection board of the elite Adolf Hitler schools, which had been founded to identify suitable candidates for the SS.

> *'The weak must be chiselled away. I want young men and women who can suffer pain. A young German must be as swift as a greyhound, as tough as leather, and as hard as Krupp's steel.'*

Adolf Hitler

When the war began, there was a shortage of experienced teachers. This meant that two or more classes had to be combined. In the rural districts, classes were increased to 45 or more pupils per class to take children who had been evacuated from the cities.

Discipline was extremely strict and enforced with corporal punishment. Pupils were expected to stand to attention when a teacher entered and give the Hitler salute. There were no school uniforms, but every child was expected to wear their Hitler Youth or BDM uniform on special days such as Hitler's birthday (20 April 1889) and the anniversary of the Beer Hall Putsch (9 November 1923), when Hitler and the brown shirts had staged a failed uprising in Munich.

The innate mischievousness and distrust of authority of young adolescents could not be suppressed so easily, however. It was not unknown for otherwise conscientious pupils to distract a teacher from setting an exam by asking a question about Hitler or the origins of the party, knowing that this would set them off on a long discourse, leaving insufficient time for the test.

Outsiders

Life in Hitler's Germany was very different for non-Aryan children.

Ten-year-old Susan Oppenheimer considered herself happy and carefree until her teachers and school friends began to behave differently towards her in the spring of 1933. Non-Aryan children were moved to the back of the class and excluded from certain lessons, including PE, but never given an explanation. Susan had been particularly good at German, but she was told that her essays would no longer be read out to the class because 'only a true German could be good at German'. Fortunately, she was able to continue her athletics training by joining a club for the children of former First World War veterans, as her father had been in the German army during the Great War. But gradually her Aryan friends stopped talking to her and she was left with only Jewish children for company. Her former friends had joined the Hitler Youth and no longer spoke to her. If they did it was only to hurl abuse at her, which hurt Susan enormously. She couldn't understand why they hated her.

Then, in the summer of 1938, all non-Aryan pupils were prohibited from attending German state schools and Susan had to enrol at a private college. There, students were taught subjects that would be of use to them if they were forced to emigrate, as many were now expecting to do. But then came *Kristallnacht* and intimidation and discrimination took on a more violent and explicit form.

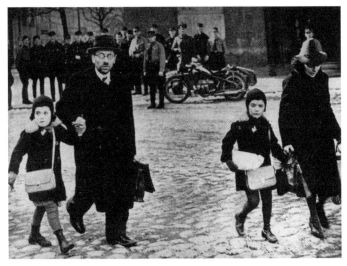

One of the first acts implemented by the new regime was the passing of a law which excluded Jews from government posts and the professions, forbade them from frequenting specific public places, such as parks, and from participating in public life and forcing them to identify themselves by wearing a yellow star on their clothes.

Susan remembered being woken that night by shouting and screaming as eight young storm troopers burst into the family home and began to vandalize everything in sight. They locked her parents in a bathroom, then attacked Susan and her younger sister. The girls were dragged out of bed and Susan's nightgown was ripped to shreds. Her parents could be heard shouting and crying but were unable to intervene. Then the SA thugs ordered Susan to get dressed, but as she opened the wardrobe they pulled it down on top of her and left, assuming they had killed her. Fortunately, it had fallen onto an overturned table, which left just enough room for the terrified teenager to crawl out and comfort her sister, who had shielded herself with blankets now covered with broken mirror glass.

The next day the family cleared up the wreckage of their apartment with the help of an elderly maid who admitted she was a staunch admirer of Hitler and who could not believe that he had sanctioned such wanton destruction.

Later that morning Susan took her bicycle to visit family friends to see if they were all right – no one dared use the phone for fear that it was being tapped by the Gestapo. All had suffered traumatic experiences the previous night. Now they urged each other to leave the city as the notorious Jew-baiter Julius Streicher was organizing a mass rally for that evening at which it was feared he would call for more attacks on the Jews of Nuremberg. The Oppenheimer family decided to drive to the British consulate in Munich but they were stopped soon after they reached the city, their father was arrested and the car confiscated. When their mother enquired when she might see her husband again she was told that they would be sent his ashes. As Susan later learned, her father was already on his way to Dachau.

Judy Benton had a similar experience as a schoolgirl in Meissen near Dresden. She too was moved to the back of the class, but had the added indignity of sitting at a desk painted yellow and inscribed: 'Here sits a dirty Jewish girl.' The teacher refused to mark her work and she was denied the first prize for coming top in her class, after being told that she had earned it. But she didn't complain when she was informed that the prize was a copy of *Mein Kampf.*

Judy remembered with some bitterness that the teachers rarely failed to find an opportunity to ridicule her. On one occasion a teacher brought in a poster purporting to explain how to identify a Jew: it listed black hair, a large hooked nose and yellowed fingers from counting money.

Judy's father had lost his business, a small factory producing household goods, after the Nazis seized it. One day she returned home from school to find the door open and her parents gone. A neighbour told her they had been taken by the Gestapo and she would be arrested if she remained. Showing great presence of mind, she took her passport, some money that her mother had hidden for emergencies and a small suitcase and joined a *Kindertransport* taking unaccompanied children to safety in Britain.

Without a guarantor to sponsor her and meet her at the other end of her journey, she was taking an enormous risk. But after she arrived at the station and was approached by weeping mothers begging her to look after their young children, she had the bright idea of buying a nurse's costume from a fancy-dress shop and posing as a nurse. It was an idea that saved her life.

American-born Frederic C. Tubach travelled in the opposite direction. In 1933, at the age of three, he was taken by his German parents from the safety of their home in San Francisco to Germany, where he met and befriended children of both Nazi and anti-Nazi families as well as several who were divided by their political beliefs.

His own father joined the party but his mother was adamantly opposed to extremists of any kind. He recalls that the Nazis shrewdly seduced every branch of society into believing that National Socialism would benefit all members of the community and made sure that they had a strong visual presence in every town. One particularly effective example was the large bright-red collection box for the poor, which fostered a feeling of solidarity within a community. Everyone, even those who didn't have much to spare themselves, contributed in the belief that they were helping their less fortunate neighbours.

For children, the big attraction was knowing they were getting 'Uncle Adolf's' approval if they excelled at sport. As an added incentive, outstanding performance in sport earned promotion in the Hitler Youth, so children began to be more aware of their grades and tried to exceed their previous best performance. Frederic remembers that he and his friends were encouraged in their love of sport by the cigarette companies that produced collectible cards of the German Olympic athletes who became their heroes.

Moulding Young Minds

'Our state ... does not let a man go free from the cradle to the grave. We start our work when the child is three. As soon as it begins to think a little flag is put into its hand. Then comes school, the Hitler Youth, the Storm Troopers and military training. We don't let a single soul go, and when all that is done, there is the Labour Front which takes possession of them when they are grown up and does not let them go until they die, whether they like it or not.'

(Dr Robert Ley, leader of the Nazi Labour Front)

When he was 13, Frederic was chosen to attend a Nazi development camp where he observed at first-hand how the Nazis moulded young minds. When the boys in his room were questioned about an incident that would have had them expelled from school, they refused to give up the guilty boy and were instead congratulated for showing solidarity. 'They weren't interested in morality or social behaviour,' he concluded. 'The message was "you can do what you want, you can let your teenage violent impulses out, it doesn't matter, as long as you do it for us"'.

He found the Hitler Youth leaders unconvincing because what they taught was 'emotional and inconsistent'. The Nazis, in his opinion, were not as well practised in control techniques as the Stalinists, who exercised control over every aspect of daily life:

'The fact that Nazi concepts were so vague and unsupported by historical facts gave licence to the fanatics to say whatever moved them, as long as it stimulated hate and prejudice. Family was more important for most of us. If the family was anti-Nazi, odds were the child would be. That's a big reason the Nazis wanted to undermine the family.'

As a result of the Reich Labour Service Law, passed in June 1935, all young men between the ages of 18 and 25 were compelled to leave home and live in work camps for six months where they participated in communal programmes such as ditch-digging and marsh-draining. At the same time, their fathers might be attending party meetings, their mother engaged in the social activities organized by the League of German Girls and their younger siblings hiking with the Hitler Youth. Far from preserving the traditional German family, as it had promised to do, the regime was actively isolating the children from parental influence and working on each family member to ensure that their loyalty was primarily to the party. Parental influence was further undermined by the knowledge that their children had the power to inform on them, if only out of pique when there was a disagreement. Children were also encouraged to take an 'active interest' in the political opinions of their parents by their teachers, who would ask them to write essays on family life and the topics discussed by their parents.

The Church at that time exerted a strong moral influence on a sizeable proportion of the population, particularly in the predominantly Catholic south, specifically Bavaria. For this reason the Nazis actively sought to undermine the authority of the Church by imposing its own neo-pagan religion, with Nazi-themed weddings and funerals in which the Bible was replaced by *Mein Kampf*, the Holy Cross by the swastika and Christ was supplanted by Hitler.

However, religious conviction prevented many devout Christians from accepting Hitler as the new messiah. Nevertheless, young men such as Professor Tubach felt at the time that the mantra they chanted at each meeting of the *Jungvolk* in honour of the Führer was intended to invest Hitler with a special aura and empower his followers in the same way that a communal hymn gives the worshipper a sense of the divine.

Professor Tubach also recalled that in camp he and his young comrades were encouraged to make as much noise as they wished while they awaited meals and at meetings – in stark contrast to the customary prayer that many would have been expected to say at home. Evidently the party wanted to subvert the boys' traditional religious upbringing in order to destroy 'moral sensibilities and civilized behaviour'.

These asocial impulses were seen as positive attributes by the authors of the various leadership manuals:

'The protection of the home and bourgeois behaviour are despised. Industriousness in school is discarded for the sake of courage and physical prowess.'
(*Geist der Jungmannschaft*, 1934)

Hitler Youth

'In my Ordensburgen ... a youth will grow up that will horrify the world. I want to have a violent, lordly fearless, cruel youth ... They have to suffer and conquer pain. Nothing gentle and weak in them must be left.'
(Hitler, *Der Nationalsozialismus. Dokumente 1939–1945*, ed. Walther Hofer)

One of the many crimes committed by the Nazi leadership for which they were not indicted at Nuremberg was the betrayal of the nation's youth. During the 12 years of Nazi rule, a generation of young people were indoctrinated with the regime's specious racial ideology, conditioned to submit to authority without question and compelled to join youth organizations that suppressed their individuality in order to create soulless, obedient automatons.

Ilse McKee was 11 years old when Hitler came to power in 1933, the year membership of the Hitler Youth increased rapidly from 50,000 to more than two million. The organization

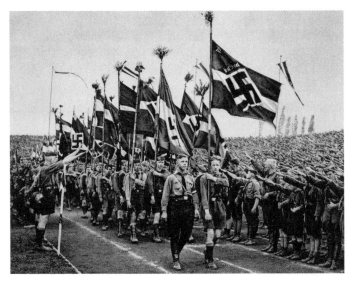

The Hitler Youth was conceived as a precursor to military service and emphasized strict discipline, order and unquestioning loyalty and obedience to the leadership.

had been formed in 1926, but regular attendance is believed to have been as low as 25 per cent until membership became compulsory in December 1936, when its ranks swelled to more than four million (90 per cent of the nation's youth).

It has been generally accepted that membership of the Nazi youth groups was compulsory, with every Aryan boy over the age of 14 obliged to join the Hitler Youth and those between 10 and 14 required to enrol in the *Jungvolk*, but it was not mandatory until 1939.

Without doubt the most popular activities for boys were the *Geländespiele* [war games], which required stealth, strategy and surprise to outmanoeuvre and capture a pre-arranged landmark from the defending team. But even this innocent children's game was adapted to encourage self-sacrifice for the common good, rather than encouraging a rational solution that achieved its objective with the minimum loss of life. It was obvious to even the most subservient, unthinking member of the Hitler Youth that their training had little to do with scouting and more to do with soldiering.

Girls were required to join the League of German Girls and its sister organization, the Young Girls, bringing total membership of the four youth groups to seven and a half million, or three-quarters of those eligible to join. But many young people had been inducted after their non-political youth organization had been dissolved and their members were automatically enrolled in the Nazi Youth groups. Even then, there were ways to avoid attendance on medical grounds or simply by virtue of having to study, which left no time for extracurricular activities.

The two female branches of the *Bund Deutscher Mädel* [BDM, League of German Girls] initially proved more popular than the equivalent male organizations because they offered girls the opportunity to participate in activities that had been considered more suitable for boys, such as hiking. In addition, they promised to teach them subjects that were not included on the state school curriculum, namely arts, crafts, music and theatre as well as the making and mending of their own clothes and basic domestic skills.

Not everyone in the Nazi leadership, however, was impressed by their newfound skills and discipline. Himmler was overheard to remark that when he saw girls marching in ranks dressed in their brown *Kletterjacke* [climbing jackets], white blouse and dark blue skirts, he felt sick to his stomach. Parents, too, had their reservations, particularly those who

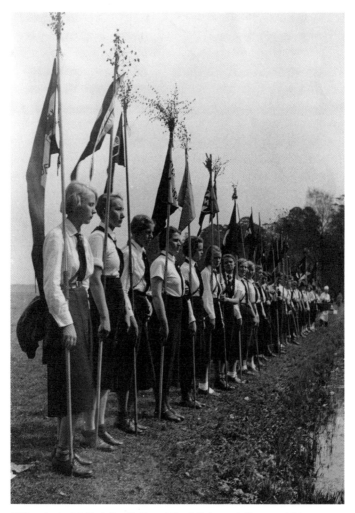

Hitler declared that the National Socialist revolution would be an entirely male event and was horrified to see women marching in uniform at the Nuremberg Rallies.

would have preferred to see their children in church on a Sunday morning rather than going on group outings.

Girls between the ages of 10 and 14 were encouraged to join the *Jungmädel* [Young Girls' League], the junior branch of the BDM, whose only qualifications for entry were proof of racial purity and a minimum standard of fitness and athletic ability. Girls were required to attend twice-weekly evening classes and to be present at every youth rally and sports event. Weekends were a continuous programme of group activities involving hiking with a full pack, scavenger hunts, camping and fund-raising events. These activities proved beneficial for physical fitness, but left the girls little time for their school work. Consequently, many failed to acquire a basic education or obtain essential qualifications. It was common for teachers to complain that pupils were too tired to stay awake in class the morning after attending an evening BDM meeting.

Evening classes were invariably taken by girls not much older than those they were instructing and consisted mainly of songs and political lectures, which the older girls taught by rote, often with little understanding of what they were teaching. In order to maintain discipline, drills would be organized during which the girls were marched up and down like soldiers on a parade ground while the *Scharfuehrerinnen* [group leaders] barked orders. It must have seemed pointless to girls of that age, especially when they were being constantly told that they were being prepared for motherhood.

Both the boys' and girls' classes would be held in the same building so that they could all attend the lectures on racial topics and the importance of raising the birth rate. Ilse

McKee recalls being unable to suppress a giggle at the thought of the 'spidery-legged, pimply little cockerels' who were expected to father the soldiers of the future. Inevitably, there were numerous unplanned teenage pregnancies, of which the boys boasted and about which the girls felt a sense of pride rather than shame, as they considered it their duty to breed babies like battery hens.

Ballot Rigging

Once the Nazis were in power they could take it for granted that the result in any future elections or plebiscites (referendums) would be in their favour. Unfortunately for them, in the March 1936 election their ballot rigging caused them some embarrassment when the result gave them exactly 99 per cent of the votes in every district of Berlin. In Friedrichshagen, 15 voting centres recorded as many votes as there were registered voters and the remaining five centres had only one vote less. As *Gauleiter* [party leader] of Berlin, Dr Goebbels was not amused and ordered a meeting of local party officials and activists at which he warned them to be more circumspect in future.

In Hamburg, ballot papers for the national plebiscite on Germany's reoccupation of the Rhineland had been numbered in invisible ink and those who voted against were subsequently arrested. Knowing this, trainee lawyer Peter Bielenberg volunteered to assist with the count in his district of Berlin later that same year – in a vote called to approve more of the party's policies – and was elated to see that many had voted 'no'. But the next morning the newspapers declared a unanimous vote in the party's favour, confirming what every free-thinking German had feared: the opposition had been effectively silenced and more severe measures would need to be taken to remove the dictator.

Chapter Three
Myth of the Master Race

Getting in Step

'It don't mean a thing if it ain't got that swing.'
(Duke Ellington)

While all of Germany seemed to be marching in step behind their leader, there was a small but significant number of non-conformists who chose to dance to a different tune. Although it took considerable courage to openly flout the diktats of a totalitarian regime, the 'swing kids', as they became known, were not particularly politically astute, nor were they all ideologically opposed to the Nazis on principle. Many were simply adolescents who were determined to exercise their right to do as they damn well pleased. They resented being told what they were allowed to wear, how to cut their hair and what music they were forbidden to listen to. The fact that they were living under the most repressive regime in modern times did not deter them from asserting their individuality and cocking a snoot at authority.

In the mid-1930s, a new form of up-tempo American jazz with a syncopated rhythm was electrifying the airwaves all around the world and filling ballroom and nightclub dance floors with jitterbugging teens. They called it swing and German youth saw no reason why they should be forced to sit on the sidelines and watch the free world have their fun. The regime had made it known that they disapproved of this lascivious 'jungle music' and its flamboyant fashions, which they denounced as ostentatious and decadent. Both were said to be part of a global conspiracy to undermine National Socialism and contaminate Aryan culture.

The music was condemned for encouraging casual sex, excessive drinking and intimate interracial relationships. So the swing fans went underground, partying in private houses and in the basements of bars and cafés while continuing to flaunt their defiance in public with their flashy dress sense and hairstyles favoured by American movie stars and the reputedly dissolute English upper class.

Boys backcombed their long hair with brilliantine as if to show their contempt for the military short-back-and-sides that was mandatory in the Hitler Youth, while the girls adopted long, coiffured hairstyles in contrast to the traditional braids worn by the female members of the BDM.

The swing kids tended to come from the middle and upper classes of German society because the clothes and accessories were comparatively expensive and the lifestyle could be maintained only by the more affluent offspring.

There were regional variations, but boys generally identified themselves by dressing in knee-length zoot suits with baggy double-breasted jackets that had wide lapels, which they had seen in photographs of American jazz musicians, with perhaps a trench coat as worn by the tough guys of American gangster films, such as Humphrey Bogart and

James Cagney. Trouser turn-ups were obligatory, as were crepe-soled shoes and a pipe or a folded foreign newspaper to signal where one's allegiance lay. A Homburg with a 'gutter crown' and 'kettle-curl' brim or a wide-brimmed fedora completed the image.

Girls copied the Hollywood fashion icons as far as the restrictions on imported clothes, shoes and cosmetics allowed. The use of make-up was frowned upon by the Nazis, who viewed it as a sign of sexual promiscuity and declared it to be contrary to the natural healthy appearance of the Aryan female, so the girls applied as much as they could and in as many garish colours as they could find. It was common knowledge that the wives of Nazi officials continued to wear lipstick, nail polish, mascara and face powder in Hitler's presence and their swing sisters didn't see why they too should be denied the opportunity to look attractive.

In open defiance of Hitler's abhorrence of French haute couture and masculine attire, the swing 'chicks' mimicked the slim, boyish, pinched-waist style made popular by Parisian models and the trouser suits that movie icons Katharine Hepburn and Bette Davis had made an essential part of their image. The Hollywood stars provided the swing girls with elegant, confident role models and were often filmed or photographed affecting a carefree pose while drawing on a long cigarette holder, which the German girls also copied in defiance of Hitler's known distaste for smoking, particularly in women.

It was not only the clothes that defined a hepcat and a hip chick, but also the street slang they used, as well as their cool, laid-back attitude and swagger – the antithesis of the strict discipline instilled into the stiff-necked Hitler Youth.

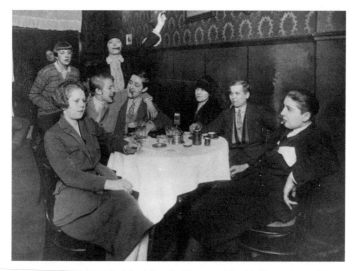

Female swing kids mimicked the fashions set by Hollywood movie icons and played with sexual stereotypes to provoke their elders and the Nazi establishment.

But the swing kids were more than a rebellious youth movement or provocative fashion statement. They were passionate fans of the music that symbolized personal freedom. The fact that it was effectively banned in Germany meant that simply listening to it on the BBC or on American overseas broadcasts was to risk arrest. But prohibition made it all the more appealing.

As records were hard to obtain and gramophones were a rarity, some swing fans made illegal copies for themselves and friends using small portable disc cutters, which put them at even greater risk. However, the majority heard their jazz in the clubs and at private parties, which were organized by someone who owned or had managed to borrow a gramophone.

For some, it was not enough just to listen or dance. They wanted to play the music themselves and soon home-grown swing bands were playing in the style of Duke Ellington, Woody Herman, Benny Goodman and Count Basie. Goebbels attempted to counter the craze by forming the regime's own rival to Basie, the innocuously named Charlie and his Orchestra, who performed pro-Nazi numbers for foreign propaganda broadcasts, but their music was as phoney as Hitler's promises.

Although there was never the possibility that a love of jazz might form the foundation for a real resistance movement, the authorities were alarmed to learn that the free form dance routines included overtly provocative gestures, such as a version of the Hitler salute incorporating Churchill's 'V' for Victory sign. Mocking the *Sieg Heil* salute was prohibited by law, so doing so even behind closed doors was a violation punishable by imprisonment. And being under the age of legal responsibility was no defence. In October 1942, 17-year-old Helmuth Hübener became the youngest of 16,500 people to be beheaded by guillotine during the Hitler years. His crime was distributing anti-war leaflets based on BBC broadcasts.

But the threat of such grim retribution did not appear to dampen the enthusiasm of the swing kids. Other seemingly innocent phrases in English or Yiddish were sprinkled into casual conversation to identify a fellow swing fan ('Swing Heil' being the most common greeting or parting phrase) or to provoke outrage from eavesdroppers and passers-by.

In 1940, the authorities attempted to crack down on the movement by installing a curfew on under-18s, but it proved almost impossible to enforce as the swing kids routinely used counterfeit identity papers to gain entrance to the clubs, bars and dance halls. Even without such papers, it was difficult to determine their true age due to their adult attire and the girls' heavy use of make-up.

The craze was so endemic in certain cities that an official report was commissioned by the Reich Ministry of Justice in spring 1944 that concluded:

'These cliques begin their activities out of a selfish impulse to amuse themselves, but rapidly deteriorate into antisocial criminal gangs. Even before the war, boys and girls from the elite social set in Hamburg would get together dressed in notorious baggy or loose clothing and become entranced under the spell of English music and dance. They often wear jackets cut in the Scot slit manner, carry umbrellas, and put fancy-coloured collar-studs in their jacket lapels as badges of their arrogance. They mimic the decadent English way of life, because they worship the Englishman as the highest evolutionary development of mankind.'

The Flottbecker Clique in Hamburg was singled out for censure by the Justice Ministry for organizing 'lewd affairs' at which up to 600 teenagers had indulged in 'unrestrained swing dancing' during the winter of 1939–40 and for openly opposing the Hitler Youth by refusing to conform and join the movement. But even after the authorities had imposed a ban on these private parties, the defiant teens continued to organize 'unlawful jamborees full of sexual mischief'.

By war's end the authorities were confident that 'evacuation methods necessitated by wartime conditions' had helped to break up these groups.

A Mixed Blessing

The swing kids were an exclusively white, middle- and upper-class clique who shared a passion for hot 'exotic' American jazz and its milder English variation. But there was one young man among them for whom the music was more than a mere adolescent obsession. Hans-Jürgen Massaquoi was a talented saxophonist whose musicianship would save himself and his mother from starvation after the war when he found employment playing for American merchant seamen in Hamburg clubs. But during the Hitler years, Massaquoi had the unique experience of being one of the few black German children growing up in the Third Reich.

As the son of mixed-race parents (his absent father was a West African law student and his mother a white German national), he was excluded but not persecuted by the regime, although he suffered racist abuse at school and at the hands of other children in his neighbourhood. He believed that he escaped deportation or worse simply because the regime didn't feel there were enough mixed-race children to necessitate a round-up.

Massaquoi was brought up by his mother to believe that he was a German 'just like everybody else' and so he couldn't understand why his teachers refused to allow him to join the Hitler Youth. He wanted to enrol so he could participate in all the activities his friends were enjoying and he admired their smart uniform.

'The Nazis put on the best show of all the political parties. There were parades, fireworks and uniforms – these were the devices by which Hitler won over young people to his ideas.'

So after nagging his mother he was allowed to enlist in a branch called the *Deutsches Jungvolk*, which brought suspicious looks from the other blond, blue-eyed Aryan boys. But Massaquoi refused to be intimidated.

As the grandson of a wealthy Liberian consul official, he enjoyed a privileged childhood in a villa on the Johnsallee and was surrounded by white servants, which led him to believe that being black meant that he belonged to the superior class. But after his father and grandfather returned to Liberia in 1929, when the boy was just three years old, his mother was forced to find work as a poorly paid hospital assistant, which barely covered the rent on their tiny new flat in a working-class district of Hamburg.

But he recovered some of his injured pride after being taken on a school trip to the Olympic Games in Berlin in 1936, where he witnessed black athlete Jesse Owens beat the supposedly superior Aryan athletes. Also that summer, American boxer Joe Louis, the 'Brown Bomber', KO'd Hitler's champion Max Schmeling in the first round of a return bout. After this, Massaquoi's classmates nicknamed him 'Joe'.

As a second-class citizen he was later excused from military service, excluded from further education and prohibited from all professions, so he swallowed his pride and took a job as an apprentice machinist. After surviving the Allied bombing that reduced most of Hamburg to rubble in July 1943, he emigrated to the USA where he took a degree in journalism that eventually led to the editorship of *Ebony* magazine.

The Berlin Olympics

'I have now seen the famous German Leader and also something of the great change he has effected ... The old trust him. The young idolize him ... not a word of criticism or of disapproval have I heard of Hitler.'

(Former British Prime Minister David Lloyd George from 'I Talked To Hitler', *Daily Express*, 17 November 1936)

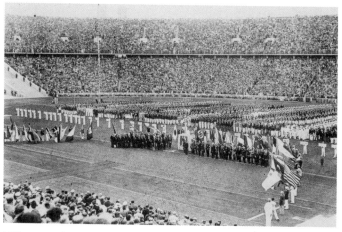

Hitler regarded the 1936 Berlin Olympics as an opportunity to promote National Socialism and prove the superiority of Aryan athletes. None of the 52 competing nations answered the call for a boycott and many teams lowered their flags in honour of the Führer as they marched passed the podium.

When Germany was given the honour of hosting the 1936 Olympic Games it was a cause for celebration throughout the country and a boost to national pride. In the eyes of its detractors, however, it served to legitimize the National Socialist revolution that was enforcing its iron rule with medieval barbarity, including torture, punishment beatings and beheadings.

Now the world's press would be invited to marvel at the changes that had taken place in the capital of the Reich and its critics would have to eat their words. That was the hope of Joseph Goebbels, who saw the games as an opportunity for the regime to showcase the remarkable achievements of National Socialism. He commented, 'Think of the press as a great keyboard on which the government can play.'

Hitler was not enthusiastic at first, but he understood the importance of the event in promoting sport among the nation's youth and also the opportunity that the games provided for the regime to prove Aryan superiority in athletics.

The Nazi leadership was so sure of success that it commissioned film-maker Leni Riefenstahl to record the event for propaganda purposes and posterity. Although her male colleagues in the industry pulled every stunt to sabotage her efforts, Hitler's backing ensured she was eventually given all the resources she required to make one of the most impressive and politically questionable documentaries ever made. In a particularly effective sequence, Riefenstahl depicted her sportsmen and women as living statues to represent the Aryan ideal of physical strength and beauty and to draw a comparison with the athletes of ancient Greece.

The decision to stage the games in Berlin had actually been made a year before the Nazis came to power, but this was brushed aside by the Propaganda Ministry at the press conference announcing the news, as were questions regarding the circumstances under which the International Olympic Committee (IOC) had reluctantly agreed to stage the 11th Olympiad in the heart of Hitler's Reich. Members of the committee had expressed alarm at reports in the foreign press of the imprisonment of political opponents and the persecution of minorities, specifically the exclusion of Jewish athletes who were well known in the athletics community. In fact, some members of the IOC were so concerned that they should not be seen to condone the regime's iniquitous racial laws that they argued bitterly among themselves and lobbied for a vote to withdraw the offer and stage the event elsewhere. The Nazi leadership was equally adamant that Germany should not be denied its propaganda coup and ordered German committee member Dr Karl Ritter von Halt to write to the IOC president denying the rumours and reports:

'Events in Germany are solely to do with domestic policies. In individual cases sportsmen have been affected. If a certain anti-German press feels called upon to deliver these domestic German matters on to the Olympic stage, then this is extraordinarily regrettable and shows their unfriendliness towards Germany in the worst possible light.'

The Reich minster for sport, Hans von Tschammer und Osten, made no apology for his country's overtly racist policies:

'We shall see to it that in our national life and in our relations and competitions with other nations, only such Germans shall be allowed to represent the nation as those against whom no objection can be raised.'

As a consequence of such statements, a number of American athletes who had qualified for the games chose to boycott the event, but they were not in sufficient numbers to make an impact.

Had America and other Western democracies taken a firm stand against fascism by withdrawing en masse from the games, it is arguable that the Nazis might have been forced to curb their programme of persecution and perhaps even reconsider their subsequent territorial demands.

Not even the German reoccupation of the Rhineland in March, nor the outbreak of the Spanish Civil War in July (which put paid to a rival event planned for Barcelona) deterred the IOC from organizing what German diarist Victor Klemperer called 'an entirely political enterprise'. And to ensure the success of that enterprise, Klemperer observed:

'The chanted slogans on the streets have been banned (for the duration of the Olympiad), Jew-baiting, bellicose sentiments, everything offensive has disappeared from the papers until the 16th of August ... In articles written in English the attention of "our guests" is repeatedly drawn to how peaceably and pleasantly things are proceeding here ... we have everything in abundance. But the butcher here and the greengrocer complain about shortages and price rises because everything has to be sent to Berlin.'

The diarist noted that the 'most loathsome' aspect of the Nazis' campaign to win hearts and minds abroad is that the state pretends to be 'an open book', but 'who chose and prepared the passages at which the book lies open? The dictatorship carries out its oppression in secret and acts hypocritically in the extreme while publicly condemning the

French Popular Front for its support of the Spanish communists. The Nazis protest, "We are not conducting a crusade. We do not shed blood either, we are a completely peaceable people and only want to be left in peace!" And at the same time not the smallest opportunity for propaganda is missed.'

The regime had learned from its mistakes in staging the Winter Olympics in February that year, when the foreign press reported seeing military manoeuvres at the site in Garmisch-Partenkirchen in the Bavarian Alps and had published photographs of anti-Jewish signs that were prominently displayed in public places. The locals had taken it upon themselves to erect these notices and had passed a bylaw prohibiting the conduct of business in Hebrew, as well as prohibiting Jews from buying or renting property in the town. Nine months before the games were scheduled to begin, the head of the organizing committee, Karl Ritter von Halt, a member of the SA, had written to the Interior Ministry to express his concerns regarding the groundswell of anti-Semitism in the area. 'I am not expressing my concerns in order to help the Jews,' he assured the Ministry, 'but if the propaganda is continued in this form the population of Garmisch-Partenkirchen will be so inflamed that it will indiscriminately attack and injure anyone who even looks Jewish.'

For the summer games, all signs banning Jews were removed, anti-Semitic posters were taken down, the military presence in the capital was reduced and 800 gypsies were rounded up and interned in a suburb of the city out of sight of the tourists. In addition, the police were instructed to disregard any minor infringements of the state's oppressive anti-homosexual laws for the duration and to keep a low profile. Behind the scenes, though, the regime refused to relax its stranglehold on censorship.

The Reich Press Chamber under Goebbels issued numerous edicts in advance of the opening ceremony to ensure that German journalists knew where their loyalties lay and what was expected from them.

They were warned not to mention that there were two non-Aryans in the women's national team or the possibility that one of them might win a gold medal in case she failed to do so.

The black athletes were not to be referred to in racial terms in case this offended the Americans and, above all, if they printed anything prior to the publication of the official and state-approved press report, they would be doing so at their own risk.

And so the 11th Olympiad of modern times opened with much pomp and pageantry on 1 August 1936, witnessed by a capacity crowd of 100,000, including ambassadors, envoys and invited guests. Among them was the aviator Charles Lindbergh, who had been rewarded for his public expressions of admiration for the New Order.

The *Hindenburg* airship flew overhead trailing the Olympic flag to an enthusiastic roar from the crowd, followed by a fanfare of trumpets as Hitler entered flanked by the officials from the Olympic Committee in their frock coats and top hats. As a military band struck up a march by Richard Strauss, the entire crowd seemed to rise to their feet en masse, raising their arms in the Hitler salute and yelling, 'Sieg Heil!'

To the evident delight of Goebbels and the other Nazi dignitaries, none of the 52 competing nations had answered the call for a boycott and the majority of the visiting teams marched past the dais lowering their flags in honour of their host and giving the fascist salute. Only the

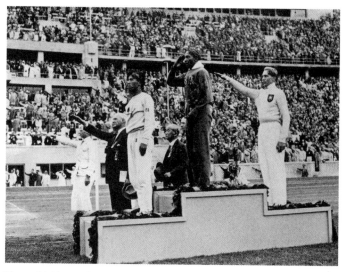

The gold (Jesse Owens), silver (Luz Long) and bronze (Naoto Tajima) medal winners of the long jump competition salute from the victory podium at the 1936 Olympic Games, held in Berlin. The Games were the first in Olympic history to be broadcast live.

Americans held their banners aloft, which drew derisive whistles from the crowd. Later the Nazis explained the slight as due to official US army regulations that forbade the team from lowering the flag for anyone other than the American president.

Goebbels declared the day 'A victory for the German cause', despite the fact that black American athlete Jesse Owens had made a mockery of Aryan supremacy in full view of the world's press. One of two Jewish American sprinters later claimed that they were substituted by Owens and another runner the day before the 4 x 100-metre relay in order to spare Hitler the sight of two Jews on the winning podium. This was denied by the coach who explained that he simply wanted to go with his two fastest sprinters.

The New York Times concluded:

'For [Hitler] it has been a day of triumph, exceeding perhaps any that have gone before. From soon after dawn, when a military parade down Unter den Linden and back revived the old imperial custom of "Great Waiting", until he retired past midnight, he was the object of enthusiasm exceeding all bounds. These Olympic Games have had an opening notable even beyond expectations, high as these were. They seem likely to accomplish what the rulers of Germany have frankly desired from them, that is, to give the world a new viewpoint from which to regard the Third Reich: it is promising that this viewpoint will be taken from an Olympic hill of peace.'

But not every journalist who went to Berlin was seduced by the obsequious smiles and the insincere hospitality. One British newspaper described the summer games as 'a Nazi party rally disguised as a sporting event', while Berlin correspondent William S. Shirer wrote scathingly in his diary on 16 August:

'I'm afraid the Nazis have succeeded with their propaganda. First, the Nazis have run the Games on a lavish scale never before experienced, and this has appealed to the athletes. Second, the Nazis have put up a very good front for the general visitors, especially the businessmen.'

Despite Hitler's refusal to acknowledge Jesse Owens' crowd-pleasing performance in public or the achievement of 13

Jewish medal-winning athletes (including a silver for German fencer Helene Mayer and a bronze for Austria's Ellen Preis), the Führer considered the event to have been a triumph. He told his architect Albert Speer that henceforth every Olympiad would take place in Berlin. (The next Olympic Games were scheduled to be staged in Tokyo in 1940, which the outbreak of war made impossible.)

Behind the scenes, however, the Berlin Olympics proved to be something of a curse for several of those who participated.

Two days after the closing ceremony, the head of the Olympic Village, Captain Wolfgang Fürstner, committed suicide after being dismissed from the army on account of his Jewish ancestry. The following year, after being denied a place in the German team, high-jump champion Gretel Bergmann fled Germany to escape the fate that befell so many of her fellow Jews. Had she been allowed to compete, it is believed she could have won another gold for her country.

But it is Owens whom history remembers as the man who defied a dictator and revealed the fallacy of Aryan superiority. He was only one of 18 African-American athletes to take part in the Berlin Olympics, however, 14 of whom won a quarter of the 56 medals awarded to the United States. Ironically, all returned home to face segregation and prejudice in their own country. Owens earned nothing as an amateur athlete and was reduced to making what can only be described as degrading personal appearances in order to secure a living.

In the last weeks of the war the stadium was used by the SS to execute 200 'traitors', many of them in their teens. After Berlin had been reduced to rubble in 1945 it remained unscathed, a monument to a time when the world allowed itself to be seduced by a regime well practised in the art of deception.

Chapter Four
Living with the Enemy

Anschluss

Austrian Kitty Werthmann was 12 years old when her country voted overwhelmingly in favour of assimilation into the Reich in the March 1938 plebiscite. For Hitler, the former Austrian corporal who claimed to have starved as a penniless artist in Vienna in the years prior to the First World War, it was a personal triumph to return to the country of his birth and be fêted as its leader.

But Kitty could not understand why a 'Christian nation' had elected such a man.

In the late 1930s, Austria was suffering from high unemployment and rampant inflation and any politician who promised to sort it out would not have been scrutinized too closely. She recalled:

'Farmers were going broke, the banks had reclaimed their farms. In the business world, they were closing up one by one. They couldn't afford to pay interest. It wasn't unusual in my home to have about 30 people a day knocking on the door asking for a bowl of soup and a slice of bread. My

*own father was hanging on by a thread. The economy was
so bad, we could almost not exist.'*

If Germany had recovered from the Depression, then it
seemed reasonable to assume that Hitler would perform the
same economic miracle for his homeland. Kitty continues:

*'He didn't talk like a monster, he talked like an American
politician. We didn't hear anything bad, about him arresting
people and persecuting people. We thought he was a
great leader.'*

On the day Hitler drove through the streets of Vienna to a
hero's welcome from adoring crowds, there was an outbreak
of Jew-baiting that made some of the leading Nazis blanch.
But it was only later that it became evident that Hitler had
returned not as a prodigal son but as a conqueror:

*'We got free radios, then he nationalized the radio stations.
We were told if we listened to foreign broadcasting we were
an enemy of the state. Then he nationalized the banks, after
he looted all the Jewish banks.'*

After the war, the Austrians would talk ruefully of the Hitler
years as if they had been occupied by an invading force and
refer to the surrender as the 'armistice', but there are those
who see no distinction between Austrians and their Nazi
brethren.

Polish peasant Stefan Terlezki was 14 years old when he
was taken from his school by the Wehrmacht in 1942 and
transported in a cattle truck to Voitsberg near Graz. There he
was sold into slavery and worked almost to death by his

Austrian owner, a farmer. He survived by scavenging potatoes, which were so plentiful that no one noticed when one or two went missing.

'Working on a farm was hell for the simple reason that as a slave you had no right to anything. You were just told, "do this, do that, come here, go there". In fact they never called me by my name, and I wondered whether I would ever be called Stefan, let alone anything else. I was called many things but not Stefan, and that was hard to swallow. Just imagine: 14 years of age and taken away into slavery. I had to look after myself. I had no shoulders to cry on, only my own.'

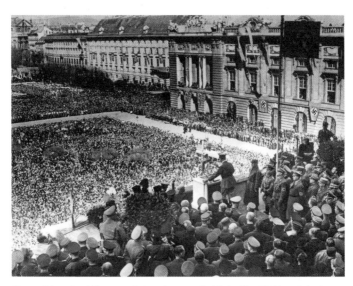

Several hundred thousand people crowded into the Heldenplatz in Vienna to hear Hitler's address from the balcony of the Hofburg, at the time of the *Anschluss* [annexation], March 1938.

Chapter Four

Preaching the Gospel

In the years immediately preceding the Nazi's accession to power, Hamburg housewife Christabel Bielenberg, who was British by birth, frequently found herself being lectured on the benefits of National Socialism by family friends and neighbours, whose intensity and dogged devotion to Hitler she found mildly amusing at first. She had become a German citizen on 29 September 1934, the same day she had married a young legal student, Peter Bielenberg, who would be imprisoned for his part in the failed July plot to kill Hitler ten years later. He would survive.

Christabel suspected that the young men she met who preached the Nazi creed hoped they might be able to convert her to their cause. But she had listened only out of politeness and curiosity. Her husband was ideologically opposed to fascism in any form and never tired of reminding her that the one time he had heard Hitler speak was in Hamburg Zoo.

Having lived in various lodgings in both the well-to-do and more modest districts of Hamburg during her student days, Christabel was familiar with the widely shared opinion on who was to blame for Germany's problems. From both the university professor that she had lodged with and the middle-class families with whom she later stayed, she heard the same arguments: the Prussian officer class had not lost the Great War, they had been 'stabbed in the back', by the Jews and the communists.

The Germans believed themselves to be the only nation that had suffered privations as a result of the war. Only Hitler understood their grievances and could bring stability and security to Germany, in the Reichstag and on the streets. He would end the violence by crushing the communists and he had promised to restore national pride by tearing up the hated Versailles Treaty and reclaiming the occupied territories taken from them after 1918. It was clear, even to a non-politically minded person such as Christabel, that this was an emotive issue and not one open to rational and reasoned debate. She found it wearisome to be harangued at every opportunity and was bemused by the ease and earnest sincerity with which they had swallowed Nazi propaganda as well as by their gushing devotion to Hitler. How could honest, hard-working Germans ever hope to get a decent job if they didn't have influential Jewish friends, they asked her. Many respectable German families had lost almost everything during the Depression. Only the Jews had thrived, she was told. Moreover, they had the facts and figures to prove it.

When Hitler became chancellor on 30 January 1933, she was pleased that these earnest people would now have the chance to see what their beloved Führer might do for Germany – she was quietly confident that they would soon be disillusioned and that another faction would be in power before too long.

But within two years the unmistakeable signs of a new dictatorship were visible in every town. Swastika flags fluttered from every public building, and main squares across the country had been renamed in honour of the Führer. The happy hikers she had once seen walking the country roads were now dressed in the uniforms of the Hitler Youth. The boys had had their hair cut short, the girls had woven theirs into plaits and many older men who had previously shown little interest in politics now sported a Hitler moustache. Individualism seemed to have evaporated overnight.

Christabel's husband found himself confronted by new requirements barring his way to his chosen profession that had nothing to do with academic ability or qualifications. All candidates had to prove their 'political reliability' and were required to submit to two months of intense political indoctrination at a semi-military camp, which would also put them through a strict physical regime.

However, for all the wariness that Christabel and Peter felt on witnessing the birth of the New Germany, it was difficult to deny that the atmosphere had changed for the better. Fear of a second financial crisis appeared to have been replaced by cautious optimism and a sense of purpose. Idle, unemployed youths who had previously loitered on street corners were now marching in smart uniforms, revealing a pride in their appearance and a gleam in their eye. Their elders were working with renewed vigour, confident that their efforts would be rewarded.

Although some had expressed disapproval of the methods Hitler had employed to purge the party of the rowdier element, it was generally accepted that the elimination of Roehm and his brown shirts on the 'Night of the Long Knives' in July 1934 had been necessary to restore order. The rivalry between the army and the SA that had threatened to erupt in a counter-revolution had been resolved and now the army was fully behind Hitler. Such unpleasantness was the price that had to be paid for the 'revolution', but now there was no more talk of dissent or pitched battles in the streets between rival political groups. And Hitler's merciless suppression of unruly elements within the SA had earned the grudging respect of the international community. Germany had regained its dignity and standing on the world stage. And everyone was once again proud to be a citizen of the Reich.

Christabel noticed that people seemed more cheerful and behaved more politely in public than before. They had regained their sense of self-worth and respectability and in return they were not inclined to question the leadership's methods. National Socialism was not so much a political programme as a secular cult that offered every loyal citizen what they had previously been deprived of – self-respect. Everyone, it seemed, had their place in the New Order and all were assured that their contribution was valued.

There was the promise of work for the unemployed, equal opportunities for everyone once the Jews had been legally excluded from the universities and professions, a level playing field for small businesses once the Jews had been forced out of theirs, long-term contracts for industry, a fully conscripted Armed Forces for the High Command, vital tasks for civil servants, prestigious titles for the bureau-crats and a new racially themed curriculum guaranteeing employment for the teachers. Even the ordinary housewife found her unpaid efforts in maintaining the home acknow-ledged and there were medals for mothers who bore the most children.

And for those lowly individuals without official status who desired to be known and to exercise power over their neigh-bours, there was the opportunity to be employed as block wardens of their apartment buildings and to play the intimi-dating role of informer.

In Berlin-Dahlem, Christabel was confronted with the fact that Herr Neisse, her gardener, now had the power to have her and her neighbours arrested on the merest suspicion of disloyalty. A careless remark or a failure to contribute gener-ously to party collections could have fearful consequences.

Herr Neisse was typical of the 'common people' who had put their faith in Adolf Hitler after losing what little savings

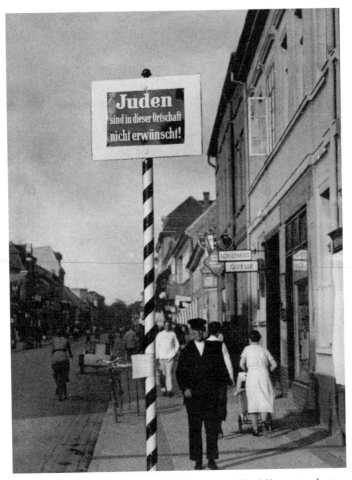

Visitors to Nazi Germany were left in no doubt that they were in a totalitarian state.

they had in the Depression. They identified with the Führer with whom they shared humble origins and modest aspirations. And they had no reason to doubt him when he identified the cause of their plight and guaranteed to make sure they had work and food for their families, if they put their trust in the party and their mark in the appropriate box on their ballot papers.

Just like Corporal Hitler, Herr Neisse had fought in the Great War and he had worked hard on his return, saving up his marks and pfennigs for ten long years so that he would have enough to marry his sweetheart. He could not understand how some had profited from the hyperinflation of 1923, brought about when Germany defaulted on a reparations payment, while he had had his life savings wiped out and been reduced to living in poverty.

He had no particular dislike of Jews but he had come to resent what the Führer had called 'international Jewry', a mythical cabal of anonymous individuals who were apparently to blame for all of Germany's ills. Whether he truly believed in this convenient scapegoat or not, it served to explain what he didn't have the education or experience to understand. Besides, Herr Hitler was so convincing it would be ungrateful to doubt him. The Führer was devoted to Germany and he must have a good heart as he was routinely photographed with small children and dogs. Who could doubt his sincerity?

But true believers, such as Herr Neisse, were stumped when asked why the Führer had signed a non-aggression pact with the Bolsheviks, who only a week before had been caricatured on party postcards wielding vicious whips over defenceless German women and children. The Führer must know what he was doing and it was not for the likes of his followers to question the leader's reasons, was the response. In the meantime, the postcards had been withdrawn only to be replaced with identical images bearing a new caption. Instead of 'Conditions in Russian concentration camps', they now carried the caption 'British concentration camps in South Africa during the Boer War'.

The fact that the conditions in British internment camps bore no relation to the vicious cruelty meted out to the starved and brutalized victims interned in Nazi concentration camps did not occur to the likes of trusting, simple folk like Herr Neisse. As for the rumours that the party elite lived in luxury in their Berlin villas and merely paid lip service to National Socialism, Herr Neisse would say only that Hitler had no knowledge of such things. It was his answer to anything that sounded remotely critical of the regime. It didn't pay to tease Herr Neisse or press him on the subject or one might find oneself in his next report.

No one was to be trusted. Even the most casual conversation with a neighbour had to be guarded and free from any comment that might be misconstrued as expressing dissatisfaction with one's lot. One could never be sure that a chance encounter had not been engineered to catch one off guard and elicit some remark that could be used to prove disloyalty to the regime.

Living under Tyranny

'Most Germans, so far as I could see, did not seem to mind that their personal freedom had been taken away, that so much of their splendid culture was being destroyed and replaced with a mindless barbarism, or that their life and

*work were being regimented to a degree never before
experienced even by a people accustomed for generations to
a great deal of regimentation ... On the whole, people did
not seem to feel that they were being cowed and held down
by an unscrupulous tyranny. On the contrary, they appeared
to support it with genuine enthusiasm.'*

(William L. Shirer, *The Nightmare Years*)

Daily life for the ordinary citizen was overshadowed by the
ever-vigilant eye of the *Kreisleiter* or block wardens who
monitored and reported any infractions to the Gestapo. Some
80 per cent of Gestapo investigations were attributed to
informers (see: Roger Moorhouse, *Berlin at War*). Germans
were, in the main, respectful of authority and adhered to
rules and regulations. They prided themselves on
Ordungsliebe [a love of order], but the presence of these local
officials soon became intrusive and intimidating. One would
routinely glance to left and right before making any remarks
that might be interpreted as critical of the regime, especially
in public places, a habit that was commonly known as the
'German glance'.

Promotion to block warden gave these individuals power
over their neighbours and many evidently took pleasure in
exercising that authority. In the province of Hesse-Nessau
alone there were 33,165 official informers on the party
payroll (see: Thomas Berger, *Lebenssituationen unter der
Herrschaft des Nationalsozialismus*).

The German writer Bernt Engelmann cites an example of
how the regime encouraged its citizens to become complicit
in its crimes. An acquaintance identified only by his first
name, Kulle, told the writer of the time his father felt he had

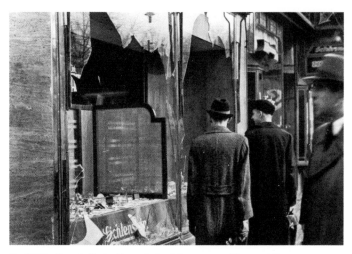

By 1938, the victimization of Jewish communities and the
destruction of their businesses was so commonplace that
many German citizens did not find it remarkable.

no option but to inform on a complete stranger to save
himself from coming under suspicion. It was the summer of
1935, and Kulle's family were staying at a hotel where the
father fell into conversation with another guest, a painter by
profession. The two men enjoyed 'very interesting discus-
sions' during their stay, at the end of which the other man
left Herr Kulle a newspaper he had been reading. It was an
anti-Nazi newspaper that had been published in Paris and
Herr Kulle feared that a pro-Nazi couple had seen him
looking at it. He had no doubt that they would report him at
the earliest opportunity, judging from the enthusiastic 'Heil
Hitler!' with which they had greeted him each morning. So he
hastily crumpled it up and affected outrage at having been
duped into reading it. His quick thinking probably saved him
as his fellow guest was an *Untersturmfuhrer* in the SS, who

immediately reported the incident to the Gestapo. The painter was arrested.

Kulle never learned what became of him, but he believed that it was only by denouncing a stranger that his father had averted suspicion from himself and saved his job and perhaps also his life.

Moral Self-Mutilation

The Nazis did not outlaw free speech overnight. Censorship came surreptitiously at first. Foreign newspapers became harder to come by. Those who trusted *The Times* to give them an unbiased account of international events, for example, found themselves making an increased effort to be first at the kiosk when the morning editions were delivered. Within a short time, news from abroad became as rare as real coffee, and there was also a risk of arrest for anyone found listening to foreign broadcasts.

The official reason for this regulation was typical of Nazi double-think. They called it *moralische Selbstverstümmelung* [moral self-mutilation], meaning the deliberate lowering of one's morale by listening to enemy propaganda. But those who desired the facts thought it worth the risk of five years' imprisonment and listened with their ear to the speaker. Even that was perilous as children were known to tell their parents that a friend had remarked that his or her mother or father listened to the radio the same way. It took only a care-less remark like that within earshot of a zealous party member and offenders could find themselves invited to explain their actions at Gestapo headquarters.

Under such circumstances, rumour and hearsay became

the main source of news. There were ludicrous tales to tease the gullible, specifically that some of the Nazi leaders were Jews (Goebbels, Rosenberg and Ley being frequently mentioned in this regard) and more sinister stories concerning what awaited those who were arrested under the so-called 'Night and Fog' decree in the newly built concentration camp at Dachau on the outskirts of Munich.

It was only when ordinary Germans were personally confronted with the consequences of the regime's decrees and directives that they understood the human cost of living in a dictatorship.

For Christabel Bielenberg this occurred the night one of her children was struck with a serious fever. Her Jewish doctor was summoned and spent all night tending the boy, which was unusual as he had previously been very busy. But she had noticed that it had become easier to make an appointment or request a house call in recent months. As the doctor was leaving that morning he asked if Frau Bielenberg wished him to continue to look after the child and when she asked why he would say such a thing, he told her that he had been ordered to close his practice and that he had received threatening letters warning him not to treat Aryan children. Instead, she was advised not to use the telephone but to come to the clinic or his apartment in person when she needed to make an appointment. The next time she did so she discovered that he had departed for Holland with no prospect of employment and that he had left all his belongings behind.

Two years later she heard from his housekeeper that he had died suddenly. Some said it was suicide, but Christabel suspected otherwise.

Her husband Peter had his suspicions confirmed regarding

the regime when he was asked to defend a Social Democrat accused of distributing illegal leaflets. No sooner had Peter offered a spirited defence that resulted in the acquittal of his client than the man was arrested under the pretext euphemistically termed 'protective custody' and bundled into an unmarked van that drove off at speed. Fruitless efforts to discover the man's whereabouts at police headquarters and the disinterested shrugs that met all his enquiries finally convinced the young lawyer that eight years of legal training had been in vain. Peter's father had worked all his life in order to be able to hand a flourishing legal practice over to his son and now it was to be abandoned. But even more disheartening was the realization that he had been defeated by a government which openly flouted the law and was in flagrant violation of basic human rights.

'Efficient intimidation can only be achieved either by capital punishment or by measures by which the relatives of the criminal and the population do not know his fate.'
(General Keitel's defence of the 'Night and Fog' decree at Nuremberg, 1946)

Sign of the Times

'No class or group or party in Germany could escape its share of responsibility for the abandonment of the democratic Republic and the advent of Adolf Hitler. The cardinal error of the Germans who opposed Nazism was their failure to unite against it.'
(William L. Shirer, *The Rise and Fall of the Thrid Reich: A History of Nazi Germany*)

If any of Germany's foreign 'friends', as they liked to style themselves – those who openly admired Hitler and defended Germany's right to rearm in defiance of the Versailles Treaty – chose to show their support by visiting the country in the years after Hitler became chancellor, they would have seen unmistakable signs that the Greater Reich was a totalitarian state.

Public parks, facilities and cafés bore signs prohibiting Jews, while other notices forbade women from smoking in public (SA men were known to snatch cigarettes from the mouths of any women caught smoking, stub them out and reprimand them for insulting the Führer, who did not approve of the habit).

Every opportunity was seized upon to demonstrate one's National Socialist zeal and allegiance to the party by imposing rules and regulations. Hotels and apartment blocks displayed notices informing residents that it was their duty to display the Nazi flag on the Führer's birthday. Many shops, restaurants and cafés put up prominent warnings to customers that the required greeting was 'Heil Hitler!' Anything other than total compliance would be interpreted as disloyalty.

The infamous Nuremberg Laws of 1935 – which deprived Jews of their citizenship, prohibited them from marrying or having a sexual relationship with gentiles and excluded them from working in the civil service and other professions – was justified by the need to 'clarify' their status in German society. A Jew was deemed to be anyone who had three or more Jewish grandparents, regardless of whether they were religiously observant or had intermarried. The measures that Hitler described as 'a definitive legal adjustment' were accepted with relief by some Jews, who hoped they might allow them to remain in Germany, albeit as second-class citizens, and that they might finally put an end to the anti-Semitic attacks, arrests and boycotts of Jewish businesses.

Night of Broken Glass

For those politicians who had hoped the 'excesses' of the regime might be reined in once they had taken their seats in the Reichstag, there was a rude awakening on the morning of 10 November 1938. The previous night, which came to be known as *Kristallnacht*, or the 'Night of Broken Glass', saw Nazi hooligans smashing shops and business premises belonging to Jews and burning synagogues in towns and cities throughout Germany, Austria and the Sudetenland. These supposedly 'spontaneous' acts of vandalism were said to be in retaliation for the assassination of a German embassy official in Paris, but they had in fact been instigated by Goebbels and orchestrated by Reinhard Heydrich, assistant to SS Reichsführer Himmler.

Some lowered their eyes and hurried past the boarded-up windows. A few expressed their disgust under their breath and hoped they wouldn't be overheard. It was a shame on the German nation and the work of the rabble. What must other nations be thinking of the Germans now? Some noted the destruction with smug satisfaction and thought that it was about time these Jews were shown that they weren't welcome. Whatever their views, from that moment on it was impossible for the citizens of Germany to deny the criminal nature of the regime. Those who naively hoped that such shameful acts might awaken those with a conscience and encourage them to take action were cruelly disappointed.

The dictatorship had a stranglehold on free speech, which was enforced by terror and intimidation. There was nothing one could do to voice disapproval.

Berlin housewife Emmi Bonhoefer was contemptuous of those who denied all knowledge of the dictatorship's persecution of the Jews and other minorities:

'Of course in '38 when the synagogues were burning everybody knew what was going on. I remember my brother-in-law told me that he went to his office by train the morning after Kristallnacht and between the stations of Zarienplatz and zoological gardens there was a Jewish synagogue on fire and he murmured, "That's a shame on our culture." Right away a gentleman sitting opposite him turned his lapel and showed his party badge and produced his papers showing he was Gestapo. My brother-in-law had to show his papers and give his address and was ordered to come to the party office next morning at 9 o'clock. He was questioned and had to explain what he had meant by that remark. He tried to talk himself out of it but his punishment was that he had to arrange and distribute the ration cards for the area at the beginning of every month. And he did this for seven years until the end of the war. The family had to arrange the cards for each category of the population, workers, children etc. but he was not permitted to have a helper. He had to go alone. That was how they broke the back of the people.'

Not everyone turned a blind eye, or lowered their gaze and acted as if nothing untoward had occurred. Johann Stab was a police officer on duty in the town of Kleinheubach on 9 November 1938, and while it is not clear from his report that

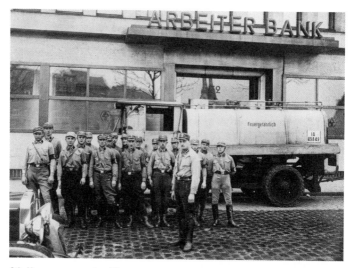

SA thugs were a familiar presence on German streets. Their actions often directly contravened German law, until the laws were changed and mob rule was legitimized.

he acted to protect the Jewish residents out of compassion, or simply to maintain law and order, it is notable that he did not allow the SA 'thugs' as he called them to intimidate him or interfere with the carrying out of his duty. When he reported the disturbances to his superior officer in nearby Miltenberg, he was told that it was not something he need concern himself with and that everything was under control. However, Stab was dissatisfied with this assurance and went to investigate.

In the main square he found that a small group of brown shirts had forced their way into the home of a Jewish resident and had begun to vandalize the property. He managed to persuade them to leave by informing them that the house had been sold to an Aryan buyer and that they were now damaging property it was his duty to protect. He was told that the group had broken into other Jewish homes and businesses and thrown furniture, possessions and goods into the street. But he was then ordered not to make arrests or to interfere. Where the order had originated he had no idea, but his superior officer was adamant that the acts of destruction had been officially sanctioned and were not to be questioned.

Later that same evening, he received further orders to take all Jewish residents into 'protective custody', but before doing so Stab locked all the damaged properties and posted an SA man outside each one to prevent further damage or looting. He then found himself arguing against the forced detainment of the female owner of a local shoe shop who was ill and confined to bed. The SA insisted that she be dragged out of her sick bed and taken to prison, but Stab was adamant that if she was to be moved at all it would be to a hospital. After much argument he managed to persuade two of them to accompany him to the woman's home where they found her clearly unwell and visibly terrified. She was 'a truly pitiful sight', sufficiently sick to convince the SA to leave her be, for the time being.

Professor Tubach, a former member of the Hitler Youth who came to despise the Nazis and after the war co-authored *An Uncommon Friendship* with a Holocaust survivor, interviewed a woman who had witnessed the aftermath of *Kristallnacht* from the safety of her classroom. She recalled that her teacher had interrupted his class to take the pupils outside to see a burning synagogue ringed with SA thugs who prevented the fire brigade from intervening. No comment was made during or after the unscheduled outing, which can be interpreted as either shameful indifference or a general feeling that the Jews had finally got what they deserved.

Jews were not the only victims of the boycott and the repercussions of *Kristallnacht*. Their Aryan employees lost their livelihoods and the older workers frequently had to take menial, low-paying jobs that crushed their self-esteem. The fact that they had worked for a Jewish business could count against them, and if they also had affiliations with opposition parties, the authorities could see to it that they were dismissed from their new post. In such cases the only option was to find *Schwarzarbeit* [illicit unregistered employment].

Political opponents, those who had been members of the banned opposition parties, were also marginalized by the Nazis. Hans-Bernhard Schunemann had been a member of the Hitler Youth, but his father had refused to join the party. Consequently, Herr Schunemann found himself demoted to technical director of his own printing firm and a Nazi was put in charge to ensure that the presses were not used to print anything that could be construed as being critical of the regime.

Goebbels' Snout

Radio, or wireless as it was called then, was a luxury until the regime introduced the state-subsidized *Volksempfänger* [people's receiver] to ensure that everyone heard the official party broadcasts. This ensured that '80 million people were deprived of independent thought,' according to armaments minister Albert Speer.

The first two-band sets sold for about half the price of

their competitors but could receive signals only from local and regional stations, ensuring that listeners could not tune in to broadcasts from overseas. The cheapest model sold for just 35 Reich marks and was popularly referred to as 'Goebbels' snout'. By 1939, it was estimated that 70 per cent of German homes possessed a radio.

The state broadcaster RBC offered a limited programme of propaganda talks interspersed with *völkische* folk music and selective classical pieces (no jazz or Jewish composers), which it was difficult to avoid as the new wireless was a fixture in many workplaces and public bars and cafés.

Both radio and newsprint journalists were vetted and their work had to be submitted to the state-controlled press agency, the DNB, for approval before publication. Criticism of the regime was forbidden as Hitler made clear in a speech to journalists on 10 November 1938:

'What is necessary is that the press blindly follow the basic principle: the leadership is always right!'

As minister for propaganda and enlightenment, Goebbels demanded tight editorial control of all publications. These included 3,600 newspapers and several hundred magazines. His memo to editors dated 22 October 1936 was typical of the thinly veiled threats he issued on an almost weekly basis:

'It turns out time and again that news and background stories still appear in the German press, which drip with an almost suicidal objectivity and which are simply irresponsible. What is not desired is newspapers edited in the old Liberalistic spirit. What is desired is that newspapers be brought in line with the basic tenets of building the

National Socialist state.'

The cinema, which had only recently found its voice after the conversion from silent to sound, was also harnessed by the regime for propaganda purposes, most effectively in Veit Harlan's inflammatory anti-Semitic melodrama *Jud Süss* (1940) and in Leni Riefenstahl's two technically impressive documentaries *Triumph of the Will* (1935) and *Olympia* (1936). The former documented the quasi-religious ritual of the annual Nuremberg Party Rally, while the latter portrayed Aryan athletic heroes as if they were gods of antiquity. However, Goebbels was shrewd enough to realize that the audience would not stand for too much proselytizing and so sweetened his message by commissioning frothy romantic comedies and melodramas that sentimentalized the self-sacrificing mother and idealized the German *heimat* [loosely, the homeland]. But outside in the real world the picture was far less pleasant.

Chapter Five
The Storm Breaks

The Onset of War

For the ordinary German, the Second World War did not begin with the hellish screaming of Stuka dive bombers and ground-shaking explosions, as it did for the civilians of Warsaw and Krakow. There were no air-raid drills or black-outs as there were in Britain, or panic buying of essential foodstuffs and petrol as there was in France, Belgium and the Netherlands. Instead, the first sign that Germany was now engaged in an international conflict came with the severing of all communication with the outside world. From the afternoon of 1 September 1939, no phone calls could be made outside of the Reich. Operators were instructed to inform callers that they were unable to connect them, but that normal service would be resumed as soon as possible.

The wireless was now people's primary source of information and all broadcasts had to be approved by Goebbels' Ministry of Propaganda and Public Enlightenment. Consequently, the tone of the first news announcements on the eve of war was one of resignation and resolve. It was 'regrettable' that events had come to this, but the leadership

had a 'clear conscience'. The German people had a right to
Lebensraum [living space]:

> **'We have done all that any country could do to
> establish peace.'**

Few who listened to the news on that mild autumn evening
would have questioned that right. For more than a year the
population of Germany and its Axis allies had been conditioned to believe that they were the victims of the vindictive
Allied powers who had imposed punitive reparations after
Germany's defeat in the First World War and who had occupied territory that the Führer had declared to be sacred soil.
The invasion of Poland was not an act of aggression, they
were told, but merely Germany exercising its authority to
'liberate' German nationals from the occupied territories and
to cleanse Europe of 'inferior races' so that Eastern Europe
could be Aryanized.

When war was declared, one of the first adjustments
everyone had to get used to was the blackout. Ordinary
blinds were insufficient, as the population was reminded in
no uncertain terms by the officious block wardens and the
police, who served a penalty notice on anyone allowing even
a chink of light to escape.

The sombre mood across the country was in stark
contrast to the drum-beating patriotism that had greeted
the declaration of war in 1918. There was also much
grumbling and discontentment, particularly in the rural
communities, which would see many older men from
peasant families – some over 40 – being drafted while a
sizeable number of young men were given exemption from

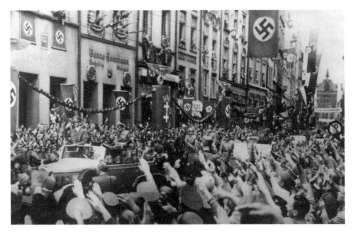

Ethnic Germans living in territories ceded under the terms of the Versailles Treaty were particularly loyal to the Führer and attracted to his policy of racial cleansing. Here Hitler is seen returning the Nazi salute to the thousands of citizens in the former free city of Danzig who turned out to welcome him.

military service on the grounds that they were in valued professions. These exceptions created a 'pervasive mood of poisonous resentment' among the population according to one official report.

But if German civilians imagined that the war would be confined to the battlefields and that early victories in Poland, France, Belgium and the Netherlands would bring peace and prosperity on the home front, they were soon disillusioned. Rationing and shortages were just two of the many inconveniences imposed on the German hausfrau in the early months of the war.

They quickly learned that the only way to acquire certain foodstuffs was either to start early and scour the market stalls for fresh produce or to ingratiate themselves with the local shopkeepers and farmers and to set aside any qualms they might have about putting the welfare of their own family before the community as the propaganda posters urged them to do. *'Gemeinnutz geht vor Eigennutz'* [community welfare before self-interest] was the slogan that reminded them of their civic duty as they joined the queue for items for which they had no immediate use, but that they thought might be necessary in the future.

Rationing was a hardship one got used to, but it was exacerbated by the fact that rations were reduced as time and the war wore on. Even the most house-proud suburban hausfrau considered erecting an inconspicuous henhouse or chicken coup in her backyard in the hope of replacing powdered egg with the real thing. And if the birds weren't productive, at least they would make a decent dinner.

In the spring of 1940, when Germans were supposedly basking in the glow of a succession of swift victories and Hitler was reported to be sightseeing in Paris, German mothers were praying that the rumours of a peace treaty with Britain was imminent so that their menfolk could come home. If asked, they would say they still believed in ultimate victory, but in the meantime they would put their faith in the black market and make do with *Sparrezepte* [economy recipes] and *Suppengrun*, a clump of vegetable stalks tied together with string that was said to make nourishing vegetable soup.

Food rationing was adequate at first but then the grocers and butchers found ways to profit by it without arousing suspicion. The easiest way was for them to tamper with the scales so that they could measure out a few grams less than the allowance. By the close of business each day the shop owner or sales assistant would have enough left over to sell or trade on the black market. Another trick they perfected was throwing the produce onto the scale and lifting it off before it could settle and register the weight. No one dared to complain for fear of being told to take their custom elsewhere.

'Guns, not butter'

The first flush of nationalist fever that had attended Hitler's succession to the chancellorship and the series of bloodless coups that saw occupied territory absorbed into the Reich faded after food shortages and the scarcity of essential materials began to hit home. The Nazis' 'guns, not butter' policy (announced by Goering in a speech he made in 1934) resulted in rationing in all but name, while the textile shortage created by the restriction on British imports in 1938 forced many Germans to face the fact that allegiance to the regime came at the cost of many basic items they had taken for granted.

Ladies were denied the luxury of imported French perfume and fashions (although the wives of Nazi officials ordered them regardless) and men found that even tailored suits were inferior to those cut from bolts of English cloth. Whereas once they could have expected a well-made suit to last for years, the German equivalent lasted barely a season, giving rise to the saying that 'German Forest' brand suits swelled in the spring and changed colour in the autumn.

Rationing was officially introduced on 28 August 1939 and limited the amount of basic foodstuffs, such as bread, flour, meat, cheese, sugar and jam, as well as shoes, soap, leather goods and coal. Even tea and coffee were soon in short supply and almost every essential item had risen in price by the end of that year.

By the winter of 1940 many German civilians were relying on handouts from the *Volkswohlfahrt* [people's welfare], the state-sponsored organization that had been founded to dispense charity to the destitute. Its Christmas package for that year contained what were already regarded as rare treats – a quarter-pound of cocoa, a kilo of lard and a handful of sweets. Some of the younger children had never seen or tasted chocolate.

By the time the Wehrmacht had suffered its first serious defeat at Stalingrad in February 1943, Germans were reduced to swapping clothing coupons for food stamps and drinking ersatz coffee – a vile watery solution made from roasted barley that reminded them of the sacrifices they were making for waging Hitler's war.

Tobacco, too, was obtainable only with special smokers' cards marked M for men and W for women, with the latter entitled to half the men's allocation. Hitler's disapproval of women smokers had apparently been circumvented on the grounds that many were now working in the armaments factories and other branches of the armed forces in a clerical capacity and needed a boost that only nicotine could offer them.

Shortages, longer working hours and drives for more productivity were largely tolerated while the German armed forces were advancing across Western Europe, the Balkans, North Africa and Russia. Imminent victory then seemed assured, but from the winter of 1942 the mood at home became considerably less optimistic. Hope of a swift victory evaporated after the shocking defeat of Rommel's

Afrika Korps at the second battle of El Alamein in November 1942. Soon after, German civilians were informed of the fate facing the once invincible Wehrmacht on the Eastern Front and asked to make further sacrifices to provide winter clothing for the Sixth Army that was besieged at Stalingrad.

News of their ignominious surrender in February 1943 was all the more demoralizing because it had followed assurances from the Ministry of Propaganda that the Soviet forces had been on the verge of collapse. But although these reversals had a significant impact on morale, it was the intensity of the Allied bombing raids on German cities that brought the gravity of the situation home to the civilian population. Each month brought more bad news that even Goebbels was hard pressed to deny, or to present as a strategic withdrawal. When news of the loss of more than 40 U-boats in May of 1943 forced Admiral Dönitz to withdraw his 'wolfpacks' from the Battle of the Atlantic, every German knew it meant that the Allied convoys would be largely unmolested from now on while their own supply ships would be at the mercy of Allied warships and fighters.

By war's end, many adults were reduced to eating horsemeat, if they were lucky enough to find it, but even starvation and the threat of being besieged on all sides failed to shake some diehard Nazis. The mood inside Hitler's Germany was grim but determined. It was summed up by a slogan that was being scrawled on the walls of bombed-out buildings throughout the country:

'Enjoy the war. Peace will be hell.'

The Darkening Storm

The mood had darkened considerably with the first Allied air raids on major German cities in the summer of 1941, and it deteriorated from then on. US correspondent William L. Shirer noted the reaction of Berliners to the first raid on the capital on August 26:

'The Berliners are stunned. They did not think it could ever happen. When this war began, Goering assured them it couldn't … They believed him. Their disillusionment today therefore is all the greater. You have to see their faces to measure it.'

But while the British were said to have pulled together and put on a brave face during the Blitz, the Germans were prone to schadenfreude, with the citizens of Hamburg and the Rhineland taking a small amount of satisfaction from the fact that it was now the turn of the arrogant Berliners to cower in their shelters under the impact of British bombs.

As time went on, however, the raids had less impact and became almost routine, to be endured like a severe winter storm. The population as a whole steeled themselves to survive at all costs and became less inquisitive about their neighbours' politics and party loyalties and more concerned about seeing it through together.

In this stifling atmosphere of suspicion and scepticism, crime flourished, despite the omniscient presence of the secret police. In the blackout, cases of rape and murder rose alarmingly, giving lie to the belief that crime would fall under a totalitarian regime. Rationing gave rise to a thriving black market in forged coupons, the theft of rationed provisions from government warehouses and general racketeering. Drug dealers, draft dodgers and other opportunists on the fringes of the criminal underworld were forced deeper underground to take advantage of a phantom economy born of austerity. This invisible population was enlarged by between 5,000 and 7,000 Jews, who were in hiding from the authorities (commonly known as 'submarines'). One such individual was Cioma Schönhaus.

The Forger

In June 1942, 20-year-old Berliner Cioma Schönhaus escaped deportation to a concentration camp because he was more valuable to the Reich as a skilled worker in one of their munitions factories. His parents and family were sent to their deaths at Majdanek extermination camp near Lublin, and Cioma was left to fend for himself. A German acquaintance had told the boy, 'It is irresponsible to pull away from the evacuation. All Jews must suffer together. All must go together. One has to obey and do what the authorities request.' Cioma's reply was, 'They can kiss my ass. I won't let myself get caught. I want to be free.'

Remarkably, in the very centre of Hitler's web, he chanced upon Germans who were willing to risk their lives to help an 'enemy of the state'. The factory foreman told him how to sabotage the machine-gun barrels that he was filing and a former government minister offered to supply him with false identity papers when it became necessary for him to disappear into the underground community of escaped Jews and other 'undesirables' living in the sewers and deserted buildings of the capital.

There Cioma survived working as a document forger, using the skills he had learned at art school to alter identity cards and passbooks for fellow 'submarines'. He also created multiple identities for himself so that he could live in a number of apartments unmolested by the Gestapo and occasionally eat in expensive restaurants that were off-limits to Jews. These included the Kaiserhof, a favourite restaurant of Hitler, Himmler and Goebbels. So he was frequently in the midst of Nazi officials – indeed, where better to hide than among the very people looking for him? He admits it gave him an adrenaline rush to defy his tormentors in this way and it became addictive.

Though obliged to wear the Yellow Star on his coat to identify himself as a Jew, he simply adapted it so that he could snap it off when entering a prohibited area and stick it back on when the police were conducting an inspection.

The ever-present threat of discovery was alleviated by his mordant humour as well as by a certain frisson he felt from playing cat and mouse with the Gestapo. After the Gestapo sealed the rooms of members of his family who had been transported to the gas chambers, Cioma prised them open, took whatever valuables he could find to sell on the black market and sealed them back up.

He also kept up his spirits by holding imaginary conversations with his dead father, who told him:

'In spite of the goods trains you must say "yes" to life. As our representative you have a duty to experience all the pleasures we were denied.'

He was aided in his efforts by Protestant members of the

Confessing Church, a resistance group who believed that it was their Christian duty to help Jews evade Nazi persecution. They would turn their identity papers over to Cioma, who would copy them for other 'illegals', then they'd claim they had lost them. They did so knowing the risk they were taking. Some were arrested and executed.

But the hardest part was simply finding a place to live. Putting on a brave front, he marched into a government office and asked for a list of landlords after claiming that he had been forced to surrender his own apartment to a relative who had been bombed out of his home in another city.

He slept at each address in turn, arriving in the evening when it was too late to register with the police and leaving first thing in the morning after claiming that he had just received his army call-up papers.

It was only when the former government minister Herr Kaufmann offered to supply him with false identity papers that Cioma decided his incredible run of luck might have been about to run out. On 6 September 1943, he packed a rucksack and pedalled across Berlin on his bike on the long ride towards the Swiss border, a copy of a book by Dr Goebbels in his rucksack in case he was stopped and questioned. A forged service record enabled him to stay in hotels and eat in cafés without attracting the attention of the authorities. He attributed his incredible good fortune to the fact that he remained unsentimental:

'When you are sad, it is like having a stone around your neck and you can no longer take action. You are lost.'

Danger and Despair

But by the spring of 1944 the average German was beginning to despair of being alive to see the end of the war. Whether it would be victory or surrender, many had ceased to care. They desired only for it to end so that they could resume their lives without the constant threat of bombardment. It wasn't only the night-time air raids that disrupted the daily routine. Every journey was fraught with danger, especially after D-Day, when the Luftwaffe were effectively grounded and the Allies were free to strafe civilian and military transport all across Germany. Some Allied pilots had become proficient at puncturing engines to immobilize locomotives, blocking the line and thus preventing other trains from getting through.

But although the structural damage to the intended targets was often minimal, the impact on German morale was considerable. Goering had boasted that no Allied bombs would fall on Berlin while his invincible Luftwaffe ruled the skies and when he was proven wrong, it gave the population cause to question what other lies they were being told.

Night after night, the Allies pounded munitions factories and aircraft engine works, and the next morning the official German broadcasts would claim that another school or hospital had been hit by the Allied 'air pirates'. But while the besieged Brits were free to turn off Lord Haw-Haw's German propaganda broadcasts, German civilians were required to tune in to folksy fireside sermons by Dr Hans Fritzsche, who urged parents to buy their children Christmas presents handmade from leather coats rather than toys, to support the fighting men on the Eastern Front. Few were persuaded – especially when faced with pleading children who didn't care a fig for patriotism.

As late as spring 1944, the German press continued to proclaim victory in two-inch-high headlines. When they finally acknowledged that their troops were making steady progress on the Eastern Front despite difficult circumstances, only the most staunch believer in the invincibility of the master race could fail to interpret it as an admission that the Russian campaign was not proceeding according to plan.

Soon every retreat became a strategic withdrawal. But the true picture of what was occurring inside Germany was to be found in the inside pages of the *Völkischer Beobachter* and its regional rivals. The implacable discipline that held Germany together under the supreme will of the Führer was beginning to crack. The unpalatable facts were to be read in the reports of the latest 'criminal' to be found guilty and summarily executed after a phoney trial for undermining the morale of the people. Invariably their 'crime' was inconsequential – the minor theft of provisions or a violation of a blackout regulation.

The message was clear: disloyalty was punishable by death.

The very thought of defeat was treasonable. And yet an increasing number of sons, brothers and fathers were coming home on leave to tell their families what they had witnessed in the east. Care-worn and weary, more than one had warned that the Russians would not be merciful after what their people had suffered under the advancing German army.

Wartime Love

While German film-makers depicted an impossibly idyllic life on the home front, not all of the country's young women

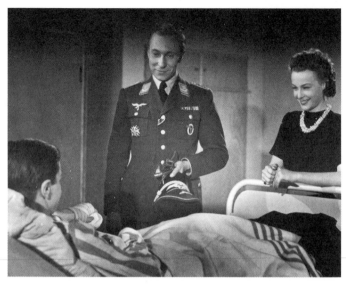

A still from *Wunschkonzert*, a hugely popular propaganda film from 1940, in which two Luftwaffe pilots fall in love with the same girl. The theme was a staple of American war films of the period and was reworked some 60 years later for the Jerry Bruckheimer blockbuster *Pearl Harbor* (2001).

suffered separation as graciously as the heroines of two of the most popular pictures of the period, *Wunschkonzert* (1940) and *Die Grosse Liebe* (1942), both of which dealt with lovers separated by the war. The constant threat of Allied bombing, the absence of their husband or lovers and the dreariness of wartime rationing and restrictions led many German women to seek the company of other men.

In the rural districts where foreign prisoners were billeted on farms, the fresh-faced symbol of Aryan motherhood often cast aside her reservations and political ideals when a suitable male companion was available, regardless of his ethnic origins. Even the threat of imprisonment was not sufficient to deter them, with the consequence that the illegitimacy rate increased five-fold in the last year of the war to 20 per cent of all registered births.

The German mother's hardship was exacerbated by the worry of having to provide for her children when there was little food to be had. But it was preferable to being separated from both her man and her child, as many were in the last two years of the war, when 1.7 million children aged between 6 and 14 were evacuated from German towns and cities under threat of Allied air attack. A further half a million children were evacuated with their mothers.

The fortunate ones found refuge with relatives, but the majority were billeted with strangers in rural areas, who resented the intruders and begrudged them anything more than the bare necessities. The city mothers tended to be seen as lazy and self-centred because many were unwilling to work as they had to care for their children, or they worked only the bare minimum for the same reason.

Berlin mother Christabel Bielenberg was acutely aware of how fortunate she was to have been offered accommodation away from the constant threat of air raids, but she was nevertheless weary of living in spare bedrooms, scrounging for food and apologizing for her children, who would misbehave from sheer boredom or because they missed their father and the familiar surroundings of home.

Some children were surprisingly resilient and resourceful, playing war games among the rubble or assuming responsibility for cheering up their mothers. One little girl knowingly exploited her starved appearance to forage for food from sympathetic farmers' wives, while a young boy found a talent for doing deals on the black market to supplement his mother's meagre income. But the majority were distressed by being separated from their parents and some were deliberately ill-treated or neglected by their reluctant hosts.

Fathers too were forcibly separated from their wives and children by the war, whether they were serving in the armed forces or working for the state in some other capacity. Some who didn't qualify for leave or who were unable to obtain it, suffered as much as their partners. First Lieutenant Werner L. from Krefeld wrote to his two-year-old daughter:

'You and your mother are going through the wonderful early stages of childhood and motherhood without me. I am still among soldiers, as I was two years ago when we knew you were on the way.'

Wunschkonzerts, the weekly forces' request programmes broadcast on the radio every Sunday night, offered the illusion of togetherness as soldiers' letters to loved ones back home were read out. These were interspersed with popular songs that they or their sweethearts and family had requested, but they were no substitute for a personal letter that could be read over and over again.

Letters Home

'As much normality as possible, as much war as necessary.'

(Nazi slogan)

During the course of the Second World War, 18 million German men left home to serve in the armed forces. For the majority of two-parent families this meant that the children were left in the care of their mother, or a female relative, friend or neighbour if the mother was unwilling or unable to give up her job. It is debatable whether this enforced separation from their husbands and partners made many of those women more independent and self-reliant. But a large proportion of the 30 million-plus letters written to and from the Home Front between 1939 and 1945 reveal that privation, suffering and the absence of a partner attested to the durability of the traditional family unit, even under such extreme conditions. And this despite the fact that 11 million German soldiers were detained in Russian POW camps for many years after the war ended. For some this extended into the mid-1950s.

The letters unearthed in the archives of the German postal service by researchers and historians are, on the whole, surprisingly lacking in sentiment and instead focus on practical advice given by husbands to their wives, encouraging them to bear up and be patient until they can be reunited. They urge their children not to neglect their school work, to help their mothers and to keep their spirits up.

The need to write and unburden oneself of pent-up feelings would not be stemmed, even when communications were severely disrupted or there was little chance of the letter being delivered. At such times many women confided their hopes and fears in the pages of their diaries. Beate K., a 23-year-old wife and mother from Königsberg, conveyed the strain of bringing up a child alone:

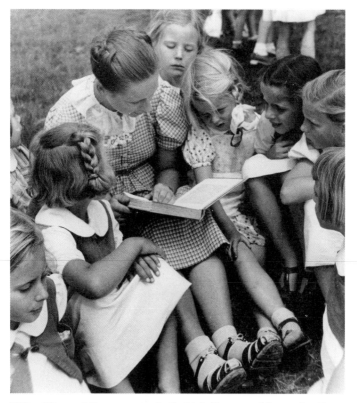

With millions of German men drafted into the armed forces for the duration of the war, children were left in the care of their mother or a female relative, friend or neighbour.

*'It would be so lovely if only your father were here ...
Sometimes it is horribly difficult to keep going.'*

Few servicemen expressed any opinions regarding the regime or the outcome of the war as every soldier was aware of the rigid censorship imposed on correspondence from the front. It was common practice for soldiers' letters to be tested for invisible ink and any form of code (even the innocuous codes used by lovers) was forbidden. The Nazi leadership was so fearful that captured German soldiers might be susceptible to Soviet propaganda that the Reich security office confiscated 20,000 letters written by German POWs, which remained undelivered at the end of the war.

Chapter Six
Witnesses

An Unconventional Family

Eycke Strickland was born in Kassel in the heart of Germany nine months after Hitler was appointed chancellor. Her 'unconventional' parents, Auguste and Karl Laabs, were pacifists on principle – her father having served in Flanders during the First World War, where he saw his older brother killed before his eyes, and Eycke's maternal grandfather having fallen on the battlefield despite his wife's fervent prayers for his safe return.

Both parents grew up to be self-reliant and somewhat suspicious of extreme nationalism. They had met through a German Youth movement called the *Wandervogel*, which instilled a love of nature in its rather idealistic members and espoused egalitarian values that Auguste and Karl in turn imparted to their children.

Karl was barred from completing his doctorate in economics and social sciences after writing a critical anti-Nazi slogan on the blackboard of a lecture hall on the day Hitler acceded to the chancellorship, and he took a job as an architect. The family settled in Wilhelmshausen, a small village north of Kassel, where Karl designed affordable houses for workers who would otherwise have been forced to live in crowded tenements.

By August 1939, on the eve of war, Eycke, her two brothers and younger sister were uprooted and moved to Vaake, another small village in Hesse, where their parents thought the family would be safer. Immediately they began preparing their small garden to grow their own food but before the planting could begin Karl was drafted to do civilian duty building airfield installations for the Luftwaffe far from home. Shortly afterwards, Auguste left the children in the care of a maid while she appeared in court to defend herself on a charge of insulting a member of the party while protesting on her husband's behalf.

But it was only the beginning of their troubles. In July 1940 Eycke's younger sister, Ute, developed pleurisy and was admitted to a children's hospital where she was treated successfully. But when the day came for her to return home, all of the children, including the contagious patients, were rushed into a bomb shelter during an air raid and Ute was infected with diphtheria and died shortly afterwards. Her parents went into mourning; her mother wore a black dress every day for a year and her father a black armband. It wasn't long before Eycke noticed that there were more women dressed in black and men wearing black armbands in the village.

However, it was not until 1941 that 7-year-old Eycke learned that 30 January had significance for someone other than her father, who celebrated his birthday on that day.

Her teacher explained that it was a national holiday because on that day eight years earlier the Führer had been appointed chancellor. At assembly that morning the hall was decorated with red and white flags and the children were told that the symbol in the centre was called a swastika. After listening to a speech extolling the virtues of National Socialism and their own privileged part as citizens of the new Germany, the class was told that they were expected to learn the words of 'Deutschland über Alles' so that they could sing it at the next assembly. Their indoctrination had begun. And yet there was something inside Eycke that prevented her from giving the Hitler salute whenever the *Bonzen* [petty bureaucrats] of the village appeared.

But Eycke's story only truly began in March 1942 when the family moved to Poland to be with their father, who was employed as the county architect in Krenau, a few miles west of a town that was to become synonymous with the Holocaust – Auschwitz.

It was in Krenau that Karl met Mordecai Hartmann, a young Jewish man who worked as a stoker in his office building and who introduced the 'unconventional' German to his family. From them, Eycke's father learned of the fate that awaited the Jews of Poland and in befriending them he resolved that he must do all he could to save as many as possible, whatever the risk to himself and his family.

For Eycke and her siblings, the 7-acre farm with its barns and outbuildings seemed like a children's paradise. They were free to play and explore, and treated the livestock as if it were their private zoo. It was only when their father erected a new fence to keep their feathered friends in and the 'troublemakers' out that Eycke wondered if it might not be the home she had always dreamed of.

No mention had been made of the previous owners, but when the duck pond was drained it threw up a short-wave radio that they must have been in a hurry to hide. Auguste ordered Mordecai to bury it and swore him to secrecy. Some time after that another incident aroused Eycke's curiosity. While out riding in an open buggy with her father she was approached by a well-dressed man who exchanged greetings with her father and then offered him a handmade Kathe Kruse doll for his daughter. The doll was much valued by collectors and would have been a rare gift for a child, but to Eycke's astonishment her father rejected it curtly saying, 'You know I cannot accept your gift. Goodbye, Herr Goldmann.' From the look on his face, Herr Goldmann was as shocked as she had been. Her father was not the kind to deny his daughter a gift from a well-meaning acquaintance and when Eycke asked him why he hadn't allowed her to accept it, he told her only, 'Eyes are watching, ears are listening', and motioned towards the driver of their buggy. The following Christmas Eycke saw her younger sister cradling it and learned that her mother had found it one day sitting abandoned on the gate post. Herr Goldmann had found a solution that did not bring suspicion on the family.

It was only much later, after the war, that her father felt he was able to tell Eycke why he had had to be careful not to be seen accepting gifts from a Jewish friend. As *Kreisbaurat* [county architect] he was responsible for issuing work permits that guaranteed food, pay and safe passage for labourers employed on municipal projects. At great risk to himself he had given priority to Jews, who were in constant threat of being transported to forced labour or extermination camps. On several occasions, dozens of the men and women on her father's list had been rounded up for transportation after a Jewish policeman had crossed their names off the list and substituted others who had presumably bribed him in an effort to save themselves. When Karl learned of it, he stormed off to the assembly area with his list and demanded that his workers be released immediately. Through bluff and bluster he managed to persuade a Gestapo official that he couldn't complete the projects without his workers and they were released.

Interview with Eycke Strickland

Eycke graciously agreed to be interviewed for this book. She asked that her answers be preceded by this comment:

'Since I am not qualified to speak for the German people, I shall limit most of my answers to what I saw and heard as a child.'

What did your parents tell you about life in Germany prior to Hitler?

Only that the years after the First World War were especially hard for my mother's family after her father was killed at the first Battle of Langemarck in Belgium. Chaos, starvation, inflation, civil unrest, lawlessness and a deep resentment on account of the Versailles Treaty reigned, as one after another the Weimar Republic governments failed to solve the country's severe problems.

It seems to me that the time was ripe for someone like Hitler, who was able to mesmerize the German people into believing that he was their saviour.

I do not remember my father sharing his views on the economic conditions leading up to 1933 with

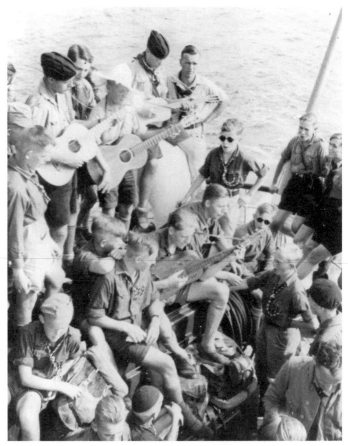

The Wandervogel - agroup of whom are seen here on an outing - together with the Bündische Jugend were referred to as the German Youth Movement. The National Socialists borrowed much from the Wandervrvogoegel, but then outlawed the groups in 1933.

me. He was more forthcoming about the political situation.

The following events and incidents are an indication of my father's attitude towards the rise of Nazism at the time:

After his return from the war, he completed his degree in architecture, and started working for an architectural firm. He became a member of a union and along with close friends shared social democratic ideals. But most of his life continued to revolve around the Wandervogel youth movement, which he had joined at a very young age, and which played a crucial role in his life before and after the First World War. He devoted his energy to rebuilding Ludwigstein Castle, which was initially dedicated to the memory of those Wandervogel who had been killed during the First World War. Die Burg became a gathering place for like-minded young men and women. My father rose to a leadership position, but resigned in 1930 because he was convinced that the new governor of the province of Hesse was imposing 'fascist tactics' in his efforts to bring the Wandervogel under the wing of the provincial government.

Around that time, my father's first marriage began to unravel. He received a scholarship from the SPD and enrolled at the Goethe University in Frankfurt.

Was there the general feeling that Hitler was the only man who could solve the nation's problems?

Again, I don't know about a general feeling, but here is what I do know:

My mother told me after the Second World War that she believed at the time that a Hitler government would not last any longer than any of the Weimar Republic Governments had. However, what many had hoped for was that Hitler's plan to get people back to work would be realized.

By chance, my parents happened to see Hitler at a small airfield as he was getting off a plane. Their reaction: 'Wir haben uns nichts dabei gedacht.' [We thought nothing of it.]

What were their initial impressions on hearing of the growing popularity of the Nazi party?

Even if the Nazis prevail over the communists in their battle over the power to rule, the Nazis aren't going to last any longer than any of the Weimar Republic governments have since the First World War.

When did you and your family become aware that the Nazis posed a serious threat to a civilized way of life in Germany?

There were many indications during the period leading up to the outbreak of the Second World War. The Nazis curtailed civil liberties, persecuted and imprisoned those whom they considered enemies of the state. Some of my parents' best Wandervogel friends were among them.

But for my father the biggest shock came when he

arrived in Poland in 1941, where he was confronted by the brutal persecution of Jews and Poles.

What was the attitude of your friends, classmates and neighbours to Hitler and the Nazis in the beginning and, if they were devout believers, did they alter their opinion to any degree before, during or after the war?

In first and second grade, my friends and I never talked about politics. Indoctrination was relatively subtle. But, I did overhear adults talking about a man named Hitler, who was getting us into trouble. Officials scolded me for not greeting them with 'Heil Hitler!'

After we moved to Poland, the indoctrination became more intense, especially in high school. All of my classmates appeared to be enthusiastic supporters of Nazism, and if they weren't, they certainly would not have talked about it.

I had one friend whose father was the director of our elementary school. He was an 'old Nazi', and when Herr Direktor Helms objected to the brutal treatment of Jews, he was tried, drafted, ordered to join a suicide squad and was killed at the Russian front shortly thereafter. I did not know what the parents of my other friends thought, and since we lived on the outskirts of town, we had no neighbours.

Even when it became clear that we were going to lose the war, the subject was taboo among my class-mates and among most adults.

My parents and their friends voiced their opinions only in hushed tones. My siblings and I were warned not to mention to anyone what we overheard or witnessed.

My general impression was that there were many people who were glad when the war was over, but there were others who had trouble dealing with the fact that Germany had lost the war and that the 1,000-year Reich had collapsed.

Uppermost in everyone's mind was to forget all about the war and to switch into survival mode.

At what point did their unqualified approval of Hitler become tinged with criticism, or did they express a sense of betrayal of the trust the German people had placed in him? Did they blame the Allies for the destruction and privations you shared, or did they acknowledge that the Nazis had brought the destruction of Germany upon themselves?

The thought of whom to blame must have occurred to them. But I'm not sure what the general public thought and felt. People were in shock, they were starving, their cities had been destroyed, they had lost family members, their men had died in battle, gone missing, were maimed or taken prisoner. Millions were uprooted and roamed the countryside looking for shelter and sustenance.

I DO know that they blamed the Allies for the destruction of their cities and the deaths of innocents due to firebombing (in Dresden).

The treatment by French and British occupation

forces of the German population was severe
compared to that of the Americans (called 'Amis').
We were grateful that we were in the American Zone.
Fear of Russian brutality was widespread. How many
people even considered that it was their revenge for
the atrocities the Nazis visited upon their homeland,
I don't know. But I do not know how many acknow-
ledged that they had brought it upon themselves by
supporting Nazism.

There were exceptions: on my website,
www.eyckestrickland.com, I cite an excellent source:

Wilm Hosenfeld, Ich versuche jeden zu retten: Das
Leben eines deutschen Offizers in Briefen und
Tagebüchern.

Here was a man who in his diary and letters dealt
with the guilt the German people had to carry.

To my knowledge, the news about Nazi atrocities
and the wholesale slaughter of millions in concentration camps began to emerge very slowly. It took
years before people started to deal with the issue.
I believe it was called Vergangenheitsbewältigung
[confronting the past].

When the war ended, especially young people
felt that they had been betrayed, misled and used.

**What was your response to the endless daily
deluge of propaganda through the radio, press
and films?**
Nazi propaganda was ingenious and very effective,
but also very puzzling. Much of it didn't make any
sense to me. Some of it sounded enticing. Some of it
was downright absurd.

I have discussed my reactions to propaganda and indoctrination in great detail in my memoir.

Did you have the impression that those you knew believed everything they were told by the Nazi leadership?

I'm sure that there were many, but not all, who did. My high school classmates certainly believed everything they were being told. If there were any who didn't, they would not have dared to talk about it.

When did you realize that the rumours of Nazi persecution of those deemed to be enemies of the state were not merely rumours?

It was when one of my brothers observed a death march and the killing of an old Jewish Oma [grand- mother]; when I heard the wailing of imprisoned Jewish families; when a boy asked my friend and me to join him at the public hanging for Jews; and when I overheard Frieda Weichmann tell my mother about the Jews 'being taken'.

More descriptions are in my memoir.

How did your father and mother explain why it was important to do all they could to save others when it meant risking their own lives and yours? What was it in their nature that was so lacking in others in that place at that time?

My parents did NOT explain anything nor ask our opinion about their rescue activities at the time. It would have been much too dangerous for us to know. It took many decades before they shared those events with us and even longer before my father decided to talk publicly about his rescue activities, and ONLY after a Wandervogel friend of the family urged him to do so. She and her husband had been members of the SPD. Her husband was imprisoned and killed during a bombing raid while engaged in forced labour.

According to professor of sociology Nechama Tec at the University of Connecticut, there is a set of interdependent characteristics and conditions that Holocaust rescuers share among them, which is the fact that they don't blend into their communities and they are independent people – and they know it. I think these best describe the nature of those who are willing to risk their lives to save others.

You have said that your father did not plan to save Jews but felt compelled to do so out of a sense of responsibility for his fellow men. Why do you think that this same sense of humanity did not compel others?

As described in Nechama Tec's academic paper 'Characteristics and Conditions Rescuers Share', it was nothing 'new or special' that made rescuers like my father decide to help the Jews and Poles who were being persecuted. My father had a history of helping others and so did my mother, albeit in a quiet, less dramatic way. If you read my memoir, you will see that my mother deserves as much credit as my father does.

In 1941, when my father became acquainted with the Weichmann family, and they informed him about the plight of the Jews, he began helping them and countless others.

He did not think of himself as a hero. In a letter to Bundespräsident Gustav Heinemann, he wrote, 'My activities during those tragic and dangerous years were for me (and my wife) only a natural act of humanness and Christian duty! Therefore, basically nothing special! It is an indisputable fact that not all Germans were passive witnesses to the Nazi terror. It was absolutely possible to resist, if one had the will and the ability to do so.'

It is entirely possible that there were many more Germans who hid and aided Jews during the Third Reich, but the sad fact remains that there are only 533 German citizens who are on record as having risked their lives and who were designated as 'Righteous Gentiles', my father, Karl Laabs, being one of the few.

You mentioned the officious types whom your father confounded with bluster and bravado, the nobodies who had been empowered by Hitler with responsibility they would never have been given in normal times. But there were also many intelligent people who succumbed to Nazi ideology. What was your impression of those people and can you explain why they too were converted to Nazism?

I have asked myself that question many times, but haven't come up with a simple answer yet. In the end, it only raises more questions for me.

Was it the ideology that attracted them?

Was it ambition, a thirst for power?

Was it their need to dominate and to feel superior to others?

It is likely that they succumbed to Nazi ideology for a lot of other reasons as well.

What would you say to those who deny the Holocaust or who claim that the entire episode has been exaggerated?

First, I would tell them of my own experiences, of what I saw with my own eyes, what I heard with my own ears and what our family experienced in a little town 11 miles from the death camp of Auschwitz.

I would urge them to look at the undeniable evidence reflected in the meticulous records kept by the Nazis themselves.

I would ask them to open their eyes to the photographs and film footage taken by the Nazis and to those taken at the time of liberation.

I would ask them to open their ears to the stories of survivors collected by Stephen Spielberg as part of his Shoah Visual History Project.

And I would suggest that they listen to the stories of some of the perpetrators, many of whom confessed to having committed unimaginable atrocities.

In the end, if all the evidence does not convince them, nothing will.

I would like to add the following narrative:

In 1948, our family like so many others at that time, were close to starvation. Some of the Jewish survivors who had been rescued by my father had been searching for us for some time. When they found us, they were thrilled. When they heard of our plight, Frieda Weichmann arrived with food and clothing.

We lost contact with them in the coming years, but when in 1983 my mother and I went to Israel to plant a tree in my father's honour, I found their addresses. We reunited with two of the sisters in Denver, Colorado, stayed in contact with them until they died and are close to their daughters and their families to this day.

During my first reading in New York, the grandson of one of the women, whose life my father had saved, introduced himself and proclaimed, 'I wouldn't be here if it weren't for Eycke's father.'

Renata Zerner

Like many Berliners, teenager Renata Zerner grew up believing that the capital of the Reich would be immune to Allied air raids. She and others reassured themselves by recalling that British and American bombers would have to fly 150 miles over enemy territory to reach the outskirts of the city, during which time they would be vulnerable to anti-aircraft fire and attack by German fighters. Besides, they had more accessible targets in the industrial Ruhr and near the coast at Hamburg and Lübeck, where the warships were built.

They recalled that Reichsmarschall Goering had given the population his personal guarantee that no enemy aircraft

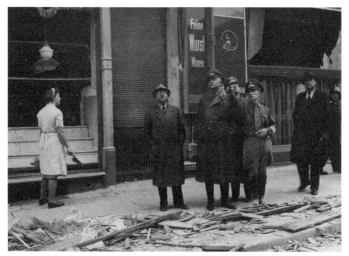

Berliners believed that the capital would be immune to Allied air raids, and that British and American bombers had more accessible targets in the industrial Ruhr and near the coast.

would get through the air defences. And yet, as early as 1940, Berlin suffered 30 raids and half as many the following year, though only two in 1942. They had all been largely symbolic, offering a morale boost for the British, and the damage had been superficial. When, in January 1943, the city suffered its first daylight raid and 200 people were killed, the inhabitants dismissed it as an anomaly, a show of force, and told themselves that if and when the raids intensified they would be targeting the Reichschancellery and other government ministries in the centre of the city, or the factories and railway yards far from the residential areas. But they were wrong.

That spring Renata was awoken in the night by sirens. She hurriedly pulled on the old clothes she kept for the long wait in the shelter. There was no communal shelter in the area and the subway stations were not as deep as the London Underground, so residents were forced to take refuge in their basements. If there was a direct hit on the five-storey apartment building in the Bayerische Platz, Renata would be buried alive with her sister Jutta and their parents along with the other tenants.

There was no ignoring the siren. Those who remained in their beds were rudely woken by the air-raid warden, a tenant who took his duties very seriously and evidently enjoyed having the authority. He would ring their doorbell until they showed themselves, then treat them to a lecture on their recklessness and lack of consideration for others, specifically himself. It was only when one of the tenants cornered him alone in a dark corridor, slapped him hard across the face and berated him for bullying them that the warden toned it down.

Berliners tend to be rather aloof, but this shared crisis brought the residents together and they began to talk more freely. While 16-year-old Renata played cards in the smaller of two cellar rooms with the other children, the adults remained in the larger room seated on an odd assortment of discarded sofas and chairs that had been salvaged from the attics. The only strangers who took refuge in the shelter were the local taxi drivers who taught the children skat, a card game they were in the habit of playing while waiting for their next customer.

The small airless room contained two bunk beds for the children, but no one could sleep on the rough blankets. In all there were about 20 people crowded into the two low-ceilinged rooms, which were brightly lit with naked bulbs.

Someone had decorated the walls with large posters of grimacing Soviet soldiers, presumably in an effort to remind them that they were fortunate to be under the Führer's protection. But it only added to their anxiety. If they survived the bombing and Berlin fell to the Red Army ... but thinking ahead was counter-productive. The only way to remain sane was to take one day at a time and believe in Goebbels' boast of final victory – which would be won with a new terror weapon that Germany's top scientists were working on at that very moment.

But such promises gave them little comfort as the sharp crack of anti-aircraft batteries grew louder and the low droning of the enemy bombers drew nearer:

'People talked in low voices, but at each blast they flinched and then they stopped talking ... A young woman, trying to overcome her fear, kept playing the solitaire she had started earlier. She dropped a card and listened. But after a moment, she picked it up and continued to play ... Suddenly, there was a whistle, and then a loud bang and the whole building shook. With one violent sweep, the woman playing solitaire pushed her cards off the table and screamed. Cries cut through the air – then stillness. My heart thumped; I could hardly breathe. Terrified, I looked at my mother, and she saw the fear in my eyes. She murmured, her face white and dead-serious, "It's all right; I think the bomb dropped very near us." My father stood up and said, "It must be the house behind us." Though he looked concerned, his voice was steady and calm.'

Renata felt safe when he was with them. Her father was a veteran of the First World War, and was fond of telling his daughters of the time he had survived an explosion in the officers' mess hall, which had been hit by a grenade. She liked to believe that his presence ensured their safety, even from falling bombs.

When the all-clear finally sounded they all brushed the plaster and cement dust from their clothes and filed out down the long narrow corridor into the street:

'What a sight! The rooftops of most of the houses around us had been hit by incendiaries, and the unchecked fires burned like giant torches. A firestorm blazed in the sky that blew the sparks into the air from rooftop to rooftop and covered the black sky with a pink cloud.'

A bomb had demolished a house directly behind them, but their apartment block had not been hit. There was little anyone could do but stand and stare at the awful spectacle. There were no fire engines to be seen or heard. There were simply too many fires for the district firefighters to cope with.

No pets were allowed in the shelter, so on returning to their apartment Renata coaxed their little terrier out from under a couch where he was shaking with fear and led him outside:

'The view was horrifyingly spectacular. Huge flames reached into the sky everywhere and caused such a storm as I had never experienced, never could imagine. It roared and howled. The fire wind tore through my hair, my eyes began to burn, and the smell of smoke penetrated my clothes and skin ... From then on, everything would be different.'

Renata's parents were anti-Nazi on principle, although her father, a physician, had been enrolled in the party by his employers, the Berlin Transportation Department, in 1933. However, after he had opened his own private practice he continued to treat his Jewish patients, although as an Aryan he was forbidden to do so, and he sustained a friendship with other opponents of the regime with whom he shared his views. To do so was to risk being overheard by informers, both those employed by the state and those who did so in the hope of ingratiating themselves with the dictatorship. Renata and her sister were warned by her parents to be discreet and not to talk politics with anyone, even with their best friends. Gestapo spies were everywhere. Storekeepers and their employees listened to customers' conversations, janitors watched the activities of their tenants and their visitors, ticket collectors on public transport eavesdropped on travellers and workmen sweeping the leaves in public parks may have been listening to casual conversations.

But even so, talking in public was less risky than sharing one's private thoughts and opinions over the telephone. Even if the phone was not tapped, Renata's parents were worried that it might have been bugged and were in the habit of putting a pillow over it when they were entertaining their 'closest friends' at home. It was rumoured that an employee of the phone company was sent to install a concealed microphone in suspect households under the pretence of checking the receiver and this listening device was capable of picking up conversations even when the phone was not being used. Renata remembers, 'We kept our doors closed and our voices down.'

Dr Zerner and his wife often met their friends on a Sunday afternoon at the Berlin Zoo in a corner where they could be sure of not being overheard:

'I learned from my parents the ability to question, never to trust implicitly those in charge, not to believe the promises made in speeches and never to ignore the atrocious propaganda posters in public places ... this kind of propaganda is designed to cause fear, and people who live in fear of a common enemy can be easily manipulated.'

Even the most innocuous phrases could be perceived as defeatist. Renata's mother was overheard lamenting the needless loss of civilian lives in an air raid and was summoned to the office of the local mayor to explain her remark. She was able to convince him that her use of the word 'kaput' may have implied that their deaths were futile, but that Berliners used that term in a different way from the people of Kassel, where she was now living with her daughter to escape the bombing.

The threat of being overheard did not, however, deter some from having fun at their leader's expense. 'What is Hitler's favourite song?' Answer: *'Ich weiss, es wird einmal ein Wunder geschehen'* [I know that one day a miracle will happen] The song had been made famous by one of Goebbel's favourite movie stars, Zarah Leander. And there was another joke doing the rounds in the last winter of the war: 'Santa Claus complained to his helpers that he was having problems finding presents for the Nazi leaders. Goebbels would be given a sexy blonde doll and Goering a toy aeroplane but there was nothing for the Führer. He had broken everything Santa had ever given him.'

But gallows humour offered only momentary relief from the grim reality of an increasingly desperate situation.

Fear of the Gestapo was very real and the merest suspicion that one might be spreading defeatist rumours would be sufficient reason for arrest.

Dr Zerner was shocked to see one of his patients, a Herr Volkmann, arrive in his consultation room one day shaking from head to foot, his face ashen and his eyes red from lack of sleep. He had just been released by the Gestapo, who had arrested him for making a derisory remark about the regime while he had been waiting in line at the post office. Herr Volkmann couldn't remember making any such remark and swore that he would never make 'political comments' in public. The informer must have mistaken him for someone else, or made the accusation out of spite. His protestations of innocence had finally been accepted as no one had come forward to corroborate the accusation. Nevertheless, Herr Volkmann now feared that he could be re-arrested at any time. But something else had unnerved him. All night he had been subjected to screaming and sobbing from another cell. When he asked the guard about it he was told it was a young boy of 17 who was to be hung for stealing a chicken.

In October 1944, even schoolboys suddenly found themselves eligible for recruitment in the SS. Dr Zerner told Renata and her mother that the SS had marched into a classroom in Berlin and ordered all of the boys to join up. One of the 17-year-olds was the son of a friend of theirs. Two months after he had been taken, he was killed on the Eastern Front.

In the final weeks of the war, neither age nor infirmity was considered a hindrance. Elderly men and young boys, some as young as 12, were sworn in to the *Volkssturm* and armed with a *Panzerfaust* [bazooka] with which they were expected to halt the Allied invaders. The population of Berlin and the cities in the path of the encroaching Soviet army were living in fear of what the Russians would do in retaliation for the atrocities committed by the SS in the east.

Elsewhere, Nazis and non-Nazis alike had learned to live one day at a time. Food had become so scarce that horsemeat was considered a luxury. Now they had no gas, electricity or hot running water. They boiled water for hot drinks and cooked by lighting fires on their balconies, if they were fortunate enough still to be living with a roof over their heads. People walked through rubble-strewn streets to work or to the market in an effort to maintain at least some semblance of normality. The shortest journey could take an hour or more. The most desirable commodity, though, was not food, but news. Every air raid brought more destruction and fresh casualties and often the only source of news of loved ones was word of mouth. Notices were pinned to the walls of shattered buildings informing anyone who wanted to know that the occupant could now be found in such-and-such a street or in the home of another family who had taken him or her in.

Renata kindly agreed to be interviewed for this book.

What had your parents told you about life in Germany prior to Hitler? Was there the general feeling that he was the only man who could solve the nation's problems?

My parents said that the 1920s, the post-First World War years, were tumultuous and difficult and the crime rate was high. The Weimar Republic was weak, and so was Hindenburg, who was old and ineffective. However, my parents often emphasized that there had been a free press and that the arts flourished. Also, going back to earlier times, they often remarked after hearing of an outrageous act committed by the Nazis, '... this could never have happened under the Kaiser'.

What were your parents' initial impressions of the Nazis?

It was obvious to them that in the beginning, almost all Germans were besotted by Hitler, and everywhere Hitler was considered the new, strong leader for Germany. My parents were Social Democrats and they became concerned about their Jewish friends, my father's patients and his Jewish colleagues.

Threats against communists, socialists, Jews, etc. intensified and were escalated by Hitler's speeches. Many Germans, as well as German Jews, assumed that it would all blow over.

Due to my young age, I really remember very little about my parents' attitudes before Hitler became chancellor except that my father would refer to Hitler and his SA troopers as 'rowdies'.

Did support for Hitler and the Nazis decline with the military's reversals of fortunes, or did the population on the whole remain staunchly loyal to the end?

I have no way to guess at even an approximate number of those who turned against the Nazis at various times, but I can say that in general, at the beginning of the war, everyone was excited about Hitler's successful 'Blitzkrieg'. But as the war wore on and people suffered from bombings, loss of lives everywhere, food rationing, etc. the support for the Nazis fell.

Please consider that in a dictatorship no one could openly ask strangers or those one didn't know very well whether or not they supported Hitler. This question could lead to interrogations or incarcerations in a concentration camp. The official opinion was: of course, everyone loved the Führer and things were going well. So why would anyone ask such a question unless he is against National Socialism?

Here is an example of the fear of being denounced:

My parents attended a dinner party given by close friends who were 'Antis', and knowing this, my mother assumed that the other guests were also 'Antis'. That was until a gentleman she had never met came to her, kissed her hand and introduced himself, murmuring 'Partei' (the German word for party). My mother was shocked and thought that he must be connected with the Nazi Party. She went to the other guests one by one and warned them not to say anything politically dangerous until she found the hostess. She asked her why she had invited an official of the party. The hostess laughed and said, 'No, no, he is all right, his name is Partei.'

One can safely assume that there were those who believed in Hitler at first and when things turned sour, they changed their minds. My mother had a good friend who really believed that Hitler meant well, but she made a quick turnaround before the year 1933 ended.

In time, Hitler's popularity did dribble down, bit by bit, but not necessarily because of the innocent victims in the camps. Mostly it was because people had to deal with their own losses, like losing family members in the war or in an air raid, or they had lost all their belongings. There was discontent in the cities that were bombed, and few escaped the bombings, and people were less afraid to make a remark in public; sometimes they burst out in frustration. Unfortunately, there were often people around who still believed in Hitler and they would turn them in. The Gestapo relied on these 'Spitzels', who were self-appointed spies. Then, after the failed assassination attempt on Hitler, the policing became stricter. It became more dangerous, and the more the German troops withdrew, the more dangerous it became. However, somehow one could feel something underneath, as if people were waiting for the end. After the capitulation at Stalingrad it became clear to many, but not all, that the war was lost.

People generally knew that there were concentration camps, but again, it is impossible to make an estimate of how many knew what really went on in them. The government's explanation was that they were re-education camps for the state's enemies. Some people found out the truth about the disappearance of the Jews, anti-Nazis, gypsies, homosexuals and others. But no one wanted to talk about what they had heard unless they were sure the other person would not turn them in.

The true believers lived in denial till the end. Our landlady and her two daughters in the little town where we lived when the bombings on Berlin increased was one of those who did not give up. After the American troops entered the town, she said excitedly, 'They are only advance troops, our soldiers (the Germans) will beat them back.' One of her daughters was a schoolmate of mine and I knew her pro-Nazi and anti-Semitic utterings well. All three of them were totally devoted to Hitler.

People in Berlin were not what in other places is considered 'neighbourly'. They greeted each other politely in the elevator or on the stairs, but there was no social talk. All that changed with the air raids when everyone went to the shelter in the basement. There we got to know our neighbours.

In the apartment house in Berlin where my family lived were eight individual apartments. Most of the renters were well educated. There was one family, all of whom were pro-Nazi. I became close friends with one of their daughters. We never touched on politics. She was a Hitler Youth leader. I was not in the Hitler Youth, but it did not change our friendship.

I want to stress again how extremely dangerous it was in Nazi Germany to ask strangers, or those one did not know well, whether or not they supported Hitler. However, there was a way to find out, and that was by developing a conversation: a vague remark of concern or by calling Hitler by his name and not 'Führer', and bit by bit one could determine where the other person stood: on the side of the Nazis or anti-Nazis.

The mentality of the Nazis is interesting. In the post-war time the fear continued, but now the tables were turned: it was the pro-Nazi types who feared admitting their pro-Nazi opinions. They thought that they would receive the same punishment that the Nazis had meted out to their political enemies. Consequently, many would not say much about their *past unless it was publicly known, and if they could, they would not admit that they had believed in, or worked for, Hitler.*

When did the unqualified support for the regime begin to crumble?

Again, it is difficult to pinpoint a specific time when the breakdown of the support for Hitler occurred, since a negative political opinion could not be expressed. After the war, much was said about speaking up or having the moral courage to stand up against the regime, but that is naive. Those who did were all killed.

It seems to me that most of the Germans blamed the Allies, certainly in the beginning. Many blamed the German people for not supporting Hitler. Eventually many realized that it had been a bad policy to invade Poland and thus start the war. And there were those who believed in a German victory to the end. For instance, our history teacher corrected us when we spoke of 'after the war'. We were to say 'after our victory'. I assume they blamed the Allies and the anti-Nazis.

Many years later, in the 1970s, a friend who had served as an army nurse in Russia during the war told me that she blamed the loss of the war on the soldiers, and that we could have won if so many of them had not deserted or capitulated. I did not ask her at the time, but I suspect that she had been pro-Hitler.

Again, at the time one could sense an atmosphere of discontent, but not much more. There were complaints about the food rationing, the lack of coal to heat the homes, lack of clothing and more. Of course, there was no gasoline for individuals who owned cars, unless they had a special need like physicians in order to make calls. In the towns and cities, people had little time after spending hours in the air-raid shelter, trying to get to work, which was sometimes impossible, or attempting to find an open food store. It was especially hard for women with young children.

No one said much aloud, but one could tell much from their exhausted looks, from their hasty, nervous manners and obvious frustrations. People from bombed-out cities who came to the small town where we stayed told each other what they had lost: their houses, or all of their belongings in the apartments. In addition, after all that, some received notice that a father, a son or a husband had been killed.

I cannot remember now, but I am sure that at the time there were people who made subtle remarks to indicate that their pro-Nazi feelings turned into feelings of betrayal. I myself feel strongly that Hitler and Nazi Germany had betrayed me and cheated me out of my youth, caused the loss of my father and my future. To know that others had lost and suffered much more never diminished my pain.

How did you insulate yourselves against the continual bombardment of Nazi propaganda?
We discussed radio, press, theatre and film at home at the dinner table. By the time I knew what propaganda was, it did not affect me. Frankly, much of it

was simplistic and stupid, loaded with slogans. I just remember one incident: I was waiting at a streetcar stop and looked at a page of the Völkischer Beobachter *paper that was posted in a glassed-in frame on a stand – obviously it was placed there for people to read while they waited for their ride. On the page was a nasty pornographic drawing of a Jew. I understood the meanness of it and was disgusted.*

The contents of most films with stars like Zarah Leander were filled with propaganda. I was more interested in the stars and their acting abilities than in the propaganda. I believe it came to a point that one did not expect anything else but propaganda. An exception was the comedies, which did not contain propaganda.

What was your impression of the effect propaganda had on your neighbours, friends and fellow students?

Many of those I knew believed everything. However, I never asked my classmates or anyone else if they believed all they were told. It would have been too dangerous. Usually they revealed their full trust, like, for instance, a woman I knew made the ridiculous comment that Hitler would invade England '... when the English Channel freezes over' (I don't know if, after the war, she ever found out the truth!).

There were others who repeated as truth everything they were told on the radio and in the press, but it's difficult to know how many and when doubts set in ... if ever. Many of the believers were badly educated, and I assume, not very bright, and much was their wishful thinking. But not all swallowed the garbage that Goebbels dished out, regardless of education.

Some very intelligent people went along with the Nazis, while some uneducated ones were against them. I think it was more a matter of gut feeling.

My family and I did not socialize with devout Nazis. If such an occasion arose, one would make small talk and, if possible, cut the conversation short.

I must have been around nine or ten when my parents discussed these matters in front of us children with the warning never, never to tell others about this 'or we would end up in one of those camps'.

When did you learn of what was happening in the camps?

We had Jewish friends and my father had Jewish patients, who told my parents what was happening. My father's office nurse (she and her family were good friends of my family) had been with us for many years, despite the Nazi prohibition to employ Jews; when it became too dangerous, she left us and later left Germany in 1939, on the day the war broke out. After the war we kept in touch with her, as well as with her surviving sister.

I was only six years old when Hitler came to power. My family was from Berlin, and Berliners in general, but not always, take a different view from the rest of the country. Being a Berliner myself, I like to think that they are perhaps more savvy in regard to politics and often better informed, since they live in close vicinity to the seat of their government and also to political gossip and rumours. What people felt about Hitler and the Nazis differed greatly in various parts of Germany, and varied depending on whether they were in the farm communities or in the cities.

The Bombing of Dresden

By February 1945 the inhabitants of Dresden were hoping that they were past the worst that the war had in store for Germany. They reassured themselves that the city, known as Florence on the Elbe because of its cultural treasures and baroque architecture, had no strategic importance and it could only be a matter of months before hostilities would cease and they could begin to rebuild their lives. But on the night of 13 February the Allies launched the first of four air assaults calculated to obliterate the city, which they considered a legitimate target because of its abundance of factories in the industrial section and its value as a communication and transportation centre.

Over two consecutive nights, 1,250 bombers dropped approximately 4,000 tonnes of high explosives and incendiary devices, turning the city centre into an inferno. The resulting firestorm caused widespread destruction and the deaths of some 25,000 civilians (the figure quoted at the time by the city authorities, which was subsequently verified in 2010, though others have claimed the number of fatalities could be far higher).

One of the survivors, Hannelore Rebstock, relived the horror of those raids in an interview with Professor Tubach of the University of California, author of *German Voices*.

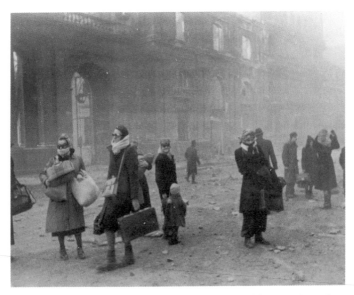

The rubble-strewn streets could make the shortest journey to and from work or school extremely hazardous, and a ten-minute walk could extend to an hour or more.

February is carnival month in Germany and the afternoon of the first air raid had seen children playing in the streets in their fancy-dress costumes, but by nine that evening, when the wireless warned of the approaching bombers, they were all safely inside their homes or tucked up in bed. Hannelore threw herself on the floor of the air-raid shelter when the first bombs fell and the ground heaved underneath her feet. As more bombs fell, the earthen floor rippled with the impact then all was silent. Hannelore and her mother emerged from their underground shelter and surveyed the raging firestorm in the company of their neighbours. It was an indescribable scene and one that has evidently haunted her ever since.

Unknown to the Allies, the population had been increased by 500,000 refugees fleeing the Russian advance, many of whom had converged on the square in front of the main railway station, hoping that they would be guided to the shelters. But the city had not built communal shelters because Dresden Council assumed that it would not be targeted. Consequently, many of these refugees were out in the open when the bombers flew over the railway station, which was a prime target.

By the time the second wave dropped their lethal loads, at around midnight, the shocked refugees had been joined by hundreds of shell-shocked residents, who had emerged from their shelters to appraise the damage. Tragically, no warning of the second raid could be given as the alarms had been knocked out earlier that evening. Hannelore survived, but she was scarred by her experience, particularly the days she spent digging through the rubble to recover dead bodies, traumatized by the sight of what she had initially thought were tree stumps, but which turned out to be the charred and distorted remains of her fellow citizens.

It was too disturbing to comprehend. She was in shock for weeks and suffered nightmares for many years afterwards. She and her fellow survivors became numb, 'dead and rigid inside'. Even while they stood side by side clearing the rubble, brick by brick, they did so in complete silence and never talked about their experience.

Anneliese Heider

During the 1930s, Anneliese Heider and her elder brother Ludwig enjoyed a typical upper-middle-class childhood in a suburb of Munich, one that offered them a singular glimpse of life in Hitler's Reich, for the Bavarian capital was the birth-place of National Socialism. Their father, Martl, a disabled veteran of the Great War, had worked as a carpenter for the railway before 1914 and on his return he was employed as a clerk. Their mother, Elisabeth, had been a cook and when food prices went sky-high in the early 1920s she still managed to feed her family by buying the less expensive offal and beef bones to make nourishing dishes.

Even after the couple had managed to save enough to purchase their newly built two-storey stucco house, they continued to live frugally, as if every pfennig counted. Martl built and repaired much of their furniture, sharpened the kitchen utensils and was proud of the fact that he wouldn't throw away a bent nail if he could straighten it and use it again. Elisabeth owned only two dresses, repaired the family's clothes and made her own pickles and preserves, which were kept in the coldest part of the hall, as fridges and freezers were a prohibitively expensive luxury.

The entire house could be warmed by a single anthracite stove, although each room had a small tiled stove that was used only when the weather was especially cold. The base-ment contained their father's workshop, the storeroom for fruit, vegetables and jars of homemade quince and apple sauce, jelly and jam. Here, too, was the laundry room where the monthly washing was soaked in a large boiling cauldron and scrubbed on a long wooden table. The wet linen was then rinsed in large tubs and wrung out by hand. If the weather was good, the damp items were hung outside to air and if not, they would be carried up to the attic where they could dry overnight.

It was an idyllic time for Anneliese with spring and

summer evenings spent playing alongside her parents in the garden, Sunday outings to the forest, visits to the circus and an annual trip to the Christkindlmarkt in Munich's Marienplatz. By the time that Anneliese was ten, she particularly enjoyed travelling into the city with her mother to shop at the big department stores. However, in November 1938 they were turned away from their favourite store, Tietz, by two brown-shirted SA men who told them, 'Germans don't shop in Jewish stores.' Anneliese was troubled, not only by the threatening presence of the SA, but also by her mother's failure to assert herself. It was unsettling to see that the people who had been turned away from Tietz had crowded into the next store and there was a long queue for the restaurant. It seemed that everyone was allowing themselves to be ordered around by the two thugs. In religion class she had been told that God loves everyone and that Jesus was a Jew. What had happened to turn her churchgoing mother and her neighbours into obedient sheep?

At elementary school the crucifix was exchanged for a framed photo of the Führer and the morning prayer was replaced by an obligatory 'Heil Hitler!' More worryingly, she was haunted by the fear of what might have happened to her new 'Sunday' friend Franz, a disabled boy who visited them one Sunday each month under an arrangement made through their church. After many happy visits during the summer and autumn of 1938, Franz suddenly stopped coming to their home and no explanation was offered. The next spring, Martl was told that Franz had been sent to a special clinic for treatment. Some time after that his family was notified that he had died of natural causes and his body cremated so that it could not be returned for burial. Two years later, in 1941, the Nazi's euthanasia programme was exposed by Bishop Galen and although the priests who printed and distributed the bishop's sermons were arrested and executed, the public outcry was sufficient to force Hitler to order it to be ended.

The war saw Ludwig drafted into the observer corps and their garden given over to growing potatoes and vegetables. As the war dragged on and rationing restricted every necessity from soap to darning thread, more of their flower beds were sacrificed for essential produce. Local produce wasn't rationed because it would spoil if not sold while fresh, but the long queues at the grocers forced many families to grow their own. Apples and pears were plentiful, but oranges and other citrus fruits were rare as they had to be imported.

German bureaucracy reached new heights of absurdity under National Socialism. Families were allowed to keep one and a half chickens per person, but these had to be registered and if a chicken died or was killed for the pot, its severed head had to be produced to prove it was no longer capable of producing eggs. If more hens were kept than the law permitted, their eggs had to be handed over to a distribution centre. Firewood became scarce but the authorities prohibited the cutting of trees or the lopping of branches, so the Heiders and their neighbours took to foraging in the woods for fallen branches after a storm. With coal a scarcity, Martl swallowed his pride and went scavenging by the railway for pieces of coal that might have fallen from the coal wagons.

Even the quality of the food changed during the war. Full-cream milk was replaced by a thin, watery concoction with a distinct blue tinge and saccharin replaced sugar. Like many Münchners, the Heider family began foraging in the woods for whatever edibles they could find. Mushrooms became a staple ingredient, but there were other sources of nourishment that served as replacements for foodstuffs and ingredients they could no longer buy. *Fichtennadelhonig* was made from the sticky new shoots of the fir tree when honey was unobtainable, and cakes had to be made with hot water and eggs as there was no fat.

Restaurants, cafés, bierkellers and hotels were also subject to rationing. Two days a week they had to provide meals without meat, and once a month many local eateries would offer a serving of vegetable stew with scraps of meat donated by the local butcher as part of *Eintopf Sonntag* [one-pot Sunday], for which customers didn't need to use up their precious ration coupons.

Anneliese confessed that what she had once considered to be necessities before the war had now become unobtainable luxuries and they had to do without them. But for children of her age there were unexpected diversions. Class would be cancelled for the morning while the children were marched to a nearby farm to pick the harmful brown-and-yellow-striped bugs from the potato plants, or harvest the crops after the farm labourers had been drafted into the armed forces. Education was no longer the priority. One of her cousins had been sent to a private school north of the city, but the students there too were excused class and sent to a hop farm where they picked hops for the breweries five days a week, returning home only at weekends.

As a member of the BDM, Anneliese was required to complete a first-aid course and her mother enrolled too, as it was evident that the population of Munich and every other town and city could no longer rely on the availability of ambulances or medical personnel after the Allied air raids intensified. And when their class finished for the day they were expected to remain and roll bandages for the front.

In the autumn of 1941, every civilian was issued with a gas mask and compelled to practise wearing it for minutes at a time. They were tight and smelled strongly of rubber. Even Christmas had to be diminished to allow for wartime restrictions. The Heider Christmas tree had been an annual delight, stretching to the ceiling, but from 1941 the family had to be content with a miniature version that stood on a table due to the potential fire hazard if the house were to be hit during an air-raid.

Despite Reichsmarschall Goering's boast that his Luftwaffe would stop enemy aircraft from bombing German towns and cities, the Allied air raids intensified through the winter of 1942–3. The Americans bombed by day and the British by night. Consequently, civilians had to be prepared to stop whatever they were doing at a moment's notice and take to the shelters. The Heider family sheltered in their own basement and made it as safe as they could from flying shrapnel and incendiaries by putting heavy cement blocks over the windows. Each member of the family packed a suitcase with essential items in case they were confined to the basement for several days and, once in the shelter, they turned on the radio to listen to the *Luftlagemeldung*, which broadcast the location of the enemy bombers.

Being in close proximity to the Dornier aircraft factory, the Heiders and their neighbours knew it would be only a matter of time before their district became a target for the Allied planes.

One clear night, the neighbourhood was roused from sleep by the wailing siren and the people rushed to their shelters, where they waited anxiously for the first bombs to fall. The noise was deafening; the ground shook and the doors and windows banged against their frames as if shaken by a fierce wind. They had been left unlocked to prevent them being blown open and causing more damage and injury. Their ordeal seemed to go on for hours but it was no more than a few minutes. However, when the all-clear was finally sounded the survivors emerged to discover that the basement shelters had not been strong enough to save their neighbours. Many houses had collapsed, burying the occupants alive under the rubble. To avoid the same fate, some families decided to build a shelter between the houses. The Heiders dug a deep trench with their neighbour and shored up the sides with timber and the roof with railroad sleepers. Several feet of sand was shovelled in on top to diffuse incendiaries and the floor was lined with old rugs. It was then stocked with water, torches, first-aid equipment, candles, tinned food and plenty of thick blankets as it was unheated. It wouldn't have been able to withstand a direct hit, but it was sturdy enough to deflect shrapnel and flying debris and that was the best they could hope for.

But still life had to go on and the population took their pleasures as and when they could. For her Christmas present that year, Anneliese persuaded her parents to allow her to go on a short skiing holiday with a friend to Garmisch, where the 1936 Winter Olympics had taken place. But even there the war was still within sight as Anneliese saw to her horror one night when Munich came under attack from Allied planes. Few homes had telephones at that time so she could only watch in shocked silence and pray that her parents were safe while the sky was lit by a fearful firework display.

When the Allies intensified their raids in January 1943, they began to use flares to guide the bombers to their targets. These lit the sky so brightly that it was possible to read a newspaper even though the city was in a total blackout. Although the military targets were now hit with more accuracy, there was still considerable collateral damage, including civilian homes, so survivors had to be rehoused. The Heider home was requisitioned for evacuees, although it turned out that these were a baroness and her daughter who had been bombed out of their palatial home in Hamburg. Having had servants to tend to their every need, they had no idea how to clean the two rooms assigned to them or cook even the most basic meals and had to ask their reluctant hostess how to do the simplest chores.

The homeless aristocrats made no concessions to their new situation, and many saw no reason why they shouldn't wear their jewellery around the house and even in the air-raid shelter.

As Anneliese grew into young adulthood she found the restrictions and wartime conditions more difficult to accept than she had as a child. She realized there were few young men to date as all but the youngest had been drafted and there were no dances to go to as public dances had been prohibited for some time. Any socializing had to be done when the weather was bad and there was less likelihood of an air raid. If fine weather and clear skies were forecast, one stayed home and waited anxiously for the siren. If the sky was overcast and there was heavy rain, it was a good time to go out to the cinema, restaurant, café or to visit friends. Daily life was turned inside out.

People dealt with the rapidly worsening situation in different ways and despite the ever-present threat of the informer, many couldn't resist a joke at the leadership's expense.

The following was typical: 'Have you heard the Swiss have

appointed a minister of the navy and they don't even have a port?' Answer: 'Well, we have a minister of justice—'

Then there was the joke about the man who showed his friend his new car. When they looked under the bonnet there was no engine. The proud owner explained, 'It's OK. I never travel to foreign countries and in Germany it's all downhill anyway.'

In March 1944, at the age of 16, Anneliese graduated and went to work in the railway administration offices where her father was employed. There she befriended other girls in the secretarial department and discovered that the war imposed further difficulties and regulations. When the air-raid siren sounded, every girl had to carry her typewriter down to the basement shelter as these were hard to replace. Just before one particular raid, several young women who were tired of carrying their typewriters up and down the stairs decided to take the elevator. Their bodies were never found.

There were 70 air-raids on Munich that year, each carried out by several hundred bombers. Few buildings escaped damage and almost every inhabitant suffered the loss of either their home, their loved ones or their friends. Some experienced all of these, but life went on.

Anneliese has given a graphic account of what it was like to be in the midst of air attack at work in her biography *Christmas Trees Lit the Sky*.

As she describes it, people were still on their way down to the basement when a bomb hit the building. As soon as the noise of the blast subsided, the air was filled with the cries and moaning of the injured and the dying. Concrete dust choked the air and rubble blocked the entrance to the shelter. There appeared to be no way out. The young secretaries clung to each other in panic, but couldn't stop themselves from shaking. Someone could be heard praying amid the pitiable moaning of the injured. More bombs struck the building and the girls looked up at the ceiling, praying that it wouldn't come down on top of them. Between the awful whistling and the impact, people could be heard calling for medics and for men to help extinguish fires that were raging on the upper floors. The girls dampened their handkerchiefs in the water buckets and pressed them to their mouths and noses so that they could breathe. Finally, the all-clear sounded and they stumbled out through a connecting door to another shelter, blindly following the person in front until they came to an emergency exit.

Outside there were hundreds of people scrambling through the rubble, searching for friends and colleagues or simply milling about in a daze.

Buildings were burning and many roads were impassable as Anneliese started the long walk home. There were no trams or trains and no familiar landmarks to tell her where she was or the direction in which she was heading. All she knew was that she had to get away from that dreadful scene. She negotiated bomb craters and walked gingerly between fallen power lines. And all the time she was trying to choke back the fear that her father had been killed and she would never see him again.

Every now and then a solitary car or small truck passed loaded with people but none stopped for her. Eventually, after what seemed like hours, she was offered a lift by the driver of a truck, who told her he was going as far as Passing, which was close to where she lived. There she was left to walk the last few kilometres past the burnt-out shells of street cars and their passengers, who would not be coming home.

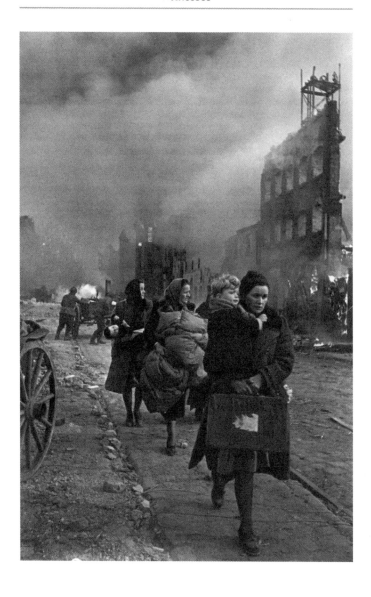

Though by now she was exhausted, once she turned into her street and saw that the house was still standing she found herself running towards it, her heart pounding, tears streaming down her face. Her mother opened the door. Her father was there too. They were all safe.

Miraculously, the Heider family saw out the end of the war in that same house, unharmed by the destruction that had raged around them.

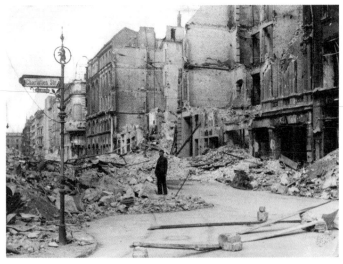

Above and previous page: The damage inflicted on German towns and cities by the first Allied air-raids did not appear to demoralize a people conditioned to expect ultimate victory, but as the raids intensified many began to doubt the propaganda.

Aftermath

After the war, Germany was invited to participate in an international cultural event, but those responsible for selecting the programme could not decide which song or piece of music would be suitable for them to perform. The German national anthem was out of the question because of its association with the Nazis, while Beethoven's 'Ode to Joy' was considered inappropriate under the circumstances. It was finally decided that the singers would perform an old folk tune, '*O du lieber Augustin*', which tells of a drunkard falling into a plague pit and emerging unharmed and untroubled by his traumatic experience thanks to the numbing effects of the alcohol. It seemed a fitting choice.

'The man who founded the Third Reich, who ruled it ruthlessly and often with uncommon shrewdness, who led it to such dizzy heights and to such a sorry end, was a person of undoubted, if evil, genius. It is true that he found in the German people, as a mysterious Providence and centuries of experience had moulded them up to that

time, a natural instrument which he was able to shape to his own sinister ends.'

(William L. Shirer, *The Rise and Fall of teh Third Reich: A History of Nazi Germany*)

Bibliography

Barnett, Victoria, *For the Soul of the People* (Oxford University Press, 1998)

Berger, Thomas, *Lebenssituationen unter der Herrschaft des Nationalsozialismus* (Hannover, 1981)

Bielenberg, Christabel, *The Past is Myself* (Corgi, 1988)

Engelmann, Bernt, *In Hitler's Germany* (Schocken, 1992)

Heider Tisdale, Anneliese, *Christmas Trees Lit the Sky* (AuthorHouse, 2012)

Hitler, Adolf, *Mein Kampf* (Jaico, 2007)

Hoffmann, Peter, *The History of the German Resistance 1933–1945* (McGill Queen's University Press, 1996)

Hosenfeld, Wilm, *Ich versuche jeden zu retten: Das Leben eines deutschen Offiziers in Briefen und Tagebüchern.* Militärgschichtliches Forschungsamt, ed. Thomas Vogel (Deutsche Verlagsanstalt, München, 2004)

Kruger, Horst, *A Crack in the Wall: Growing Up Under Hitler* (Fromm International, 1966)

Large, David Clay, *Nazi Games: The Olympics of 1936* (W.W. Norton, 2007)

Massaquoi, Hans-Jürgen, *Destined to Witness: Growing Up Black in Nazi Germany* (Harper Collins, 2009)

Mayer, Milton, *They Thought They were Free* (University of Chicago Press, 2013)

McKee, Ilse, *Tomorrow the World* (J.M. Dent and Sons, 1960)

Moorhouse, Roger, *Berlin at War: Life and Death in Hitler's Capital, 1939–45* (Vintage, 2011)

Roland, Paul, *The Nuremberg Trials: The Nazis and Their Crimes Against Humanity* (Arcturus, 2012)

Roland, Paul, *Nazi Women: The Attraction of Evil* (Arcturus, 2014)

Schönhaus, Cioma, *The Forger* (Granta, 2008)

Shirer, William L., *The Rise and Fall of teh Third Reich: A History of Nazi Germany* (Arrow, 1991)

Shirer, William L., *Berlin Diary* (Sunburst, 1997)

Shirer, William L., *The Nightmare Years, 1930–1940* (Little Brown, 1984)

Strickland, Eycke, *Eyes are Watching, Ears are Listening: Growing Up in Nazi Germany, 1933–1946.* A Memoir by Eycke Strickland (iUniverse, 2008)

Tubach, Frederic C., *German Voices* (University of California Press, 2011)

Vaizey, Hester, *Surviving Hitler's War: Family Life in Germany: 1939–48* (Palgrave, 2010)

Resources

Transdiffusion.org

Return2style.de

tikkun.org

historynet.org

theguardian.com/uk

rijo.homepage.t-online.de

nptelegraph.com

eyckestrickland.com

renatazerner.com

'The Nazis: A Warning from History' (BBC, 1997)

'The World At War – Inside The Reich' (ITV, 1973–4)

Index

Index

Index

Index

Index

Picture Credits